LIVE TO
101

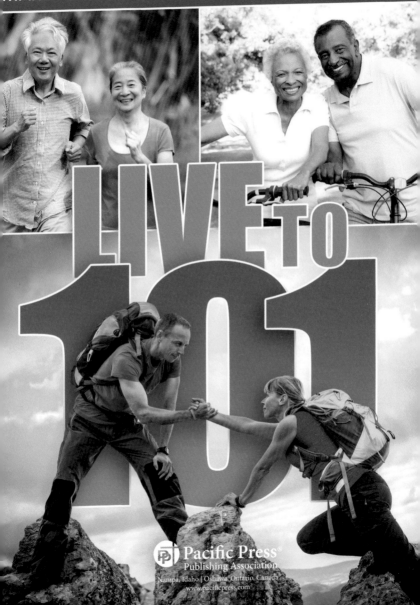

MARK A. FINLEY AND PETER N. LANDLESS, EDITORS

LIVE TO 101

Pacific Press®
Publishing Association
Nampa, Idaho | Oshawa, Ontario, Canada
www.pacificpress.com

Cover design by Gerald Lee Monks
Cover resources from iStockphoto.com
Interior design by Kristin Hansen-Mellish

Copyright © 2015 by Pacific Press® Publishing Association
Printed in the United States of America
All rights reserved.

Additional copies of this book can be obtained by calling toll-free 1-800-765-6955 or by visiting http://www.adventistbookcenter.com.

ISBN 978-0-8163-6097-0

October 2015

CONTENTS

Chapter	1	The Joy of Healthy Living	7
Chapter	2	Diet for a Lifetime	13
Chapter	3	Are You at Risk?	20
Chapter	4	Fit for Life	28
Chapter	5	Invigorated by Air, Water, and Sunshine	36
Chapter	6	Healthy Relationships	47
Chapter	7	You Are What You Think	53
Chapter	8	Hope Beyond Depression	59
Chapter	9	Breaking Free	66
Chapter	10	Rest for Our Restlessness	74
Chapter	11	The Healing Power of Faith	82

THE JOY OF HEALTHY LIVING

*More and more, people are realizing that life is best
when it's lived fully, from beginning to end.*

When Elsa Bailey blew out the candles on her birthday cake, she made a wish that she could go downhill snow skiing. And faster than you can say "Let it snow!" Elsa turned that wish into a reality. She packed her bags and headed to Keystone, Colorado, where she whooshed down the slopes, invigorated by the fresh powder and crisp air.

Turns out, when it came to that birthday wish, the only thing more strenuous than skiing was blowing out the birthday candles. There were one hundred of them after all. But turning a century old doesn't stop Elsa from living to the fullest. She has a bucket list, and the thought of, well, "kicking the bucket" isn't getting in the way of her checking things off that list.

In fact, when the local news heard about her birthday adventure, they included her story in the evening news. During the interview, Elsa was asked what's next on her bucket list, and without hesitation, she proclaimed her desire to see polar bears in the wild. Coincidentally, one of the people who saw that news report had been skiing the same slopes as Elsa that day—and she just so happened to be an employee of an adventure company that helps organize polar bear tours.

And just like that, Elsa was set to cross another thing off her bucket list. The adventure company surprised Elsa with a week-long trip to Manitoba, where she not only spotted polar bears, but also sledded with a professional dog musher—tearing through the snowy woods with squeals of delight.

Elsa has no intention of slowing down anytime soon. Yellowstone National Park is next on her bucket list, and she wants to be in good shape so she doesn't miss a thing.

When asked the secret to her long, full life, Elsa's advice is as practical as her life is fanciful: "Be active. I do things my way, like skiing when I'm 100. . . . And I try to eat pretty correctly, and get exercise and fresh air and sunshine." And don't forget to stay positive, she says, "Just smile. They say laughter is the best medicine."[1]

Life Without Limits

Elsa isn't the only one determined to pack her days with adventure and meaningful experiences. More and more, people are realizing that life is best when it's lived fully, from beginning to end. Take Anne Lorimore, an eighty-five-year-old great-grandmother, who recently climbed Mount Kilimanjaro[2]—a feat that most people one-fourth her age would struggle to complete. And then there's musician Smoky Dawson, who released an album of original songs at the age of 92.[3] And, a lover of learning, Heinz Wenderoth, DS, finished his dissertation and was awarded a doctorate degree at the age of 97.[4]

While the accomplishments of these senior overachievers may seem unattainable, the truth is, most of us are capable of achieving far higher levels of health and activity than we currently have. Just a few decades into life, many people settle in to a trance-like routine of *surviving* rather than *thriving*: drive to work, pay the bills, pick up the kids, do the laundry, mow the lawn. And, as the years pass, energy levels drop and body weight increases—making a life of adventure seem like something to watch on TV, not live for yourself.

The Happiness Lottery

Fortunately, no matter your age or health level, life can be a joy, not just a chore. Massive research confirms what you likely already know deep in your bones: you have the power to make choices that will drastically improve your quality of life.

But, let's be honest, for some people, a healthy lifestyle brings to mind dreary images of eating green leaves and dragging themselves on a treadmill in a stuffy gym. Let me stop you right there. A healthy life has gotten an undeserved bad reputation and need not be thought of as drudgery. When viewed from the right perspective, the elements of a healthy life are appealing, not dreadful. A life of motion, laughter, loving relationships, nourishing foods, sunshine, deep breaths, restorative rest, and prayers of thanks—what's not to love about that!

In fact, having good health is like winning the happiness lottery, according to a study based on data gathered by the US Census Bureau. The findings show that health is a far more powerful determinant of an individual's happiness than any other aspect of life, including income or marital status.

If you've ever thought that more money is what you need to have a happier life, this study suggests differently. Individuals in the highest income bracket—think of them as the super wealthy—are only 3.5 percent happier than average. Compare that to people who describe themselves as healthy, who are 20 percent happier than average. That means health has five to six times more impact on overall happiness than even the largest bank accounts![5]

The Power of Simple Things

Sure, the thought of a vibrant, active life can be appealing—but it can also be overwhelming. When it comes to a major health makeover, though, never underestimate the power of small, steady changes.

What difference can small things really make? A lot, according to research. One cigarette, for example, shortens your life by eleven minutes.[6] For longtime smokers, that's as much as ten years of life up in smokes.

What about something as seemingly harmless as relaxing and watching a television show? According to an analysis of Australian lifestyle data, every hour spent watching television lowers life expectancy by nearly twenty-two minutes.[7] Thus, people who watch an average of six hours a day may lose nearly five years of life compared with those who don't watch television.

The good news is that the power of small things can also work in our favor. For instance, according to one study, for every minute you exercise, you add seven minutes to your life.[8] Another study calculates that taking a twenty-five-minute walk every day will lengthen your life expectancy by seven years.[9]

All of this research confirms that we improve health the same way we take a journey: one step at a time. As you take steps in the right direction—small, healthy changes throughout your day—you'll move closer and closer to your big goals. And, before you know it, you'll look around and realize just how far you've come.

Everything Is Connected

Ultimately, health is about more than just diet and exercise. It's about the whole person—mind, body, and spirit. Science and religion agree: we humans are intricate creatures, and every aspect of us is interconnected. No surprise, then, that an improvement in one area of our mental, physical, or spiritual health brings improvements in other areas as well. That's why, for example, exercise doesn't just make us slimmer and stronger, but it also makes us happier and more relaxed, energetic, and self-confident.[10]

Throughout this book, you'll find suggestions and encouragement about how to improve your overall health and wellness. Every recommendation—from eating more plants to volunteering in your community—is a proven way to add more quality *and* more quantity to your years of life.

So, go ahead, start dreaming about all the things you want in life. Whether your heart's desire is to find more happiness and purpose, to watch your grandchildren grow up, or to experience energizing adventures and restorative rest—good health can help you get there.

You were made for this—for health and wholeness. Your mind, body, and spirit do their best work when they're being stretched to new limits, so don't hesitate to try new things. Even though aging is inevitable, you don't have to resign yourself to a miserable, limited existence. Life is meant to be lived—fully, wholeheartedly, from beginning to end.

1. Eliza Murphy, "100-Year-Old Woman Celebrates Birthday Skiing," ABCNews.go .com, May 15, 2013, accessed October 14, 2015, http://abcnews.go.com/blogs/headlines /2013/05/100-year-old-woman-celebrates-birthday-skiing/.

2. Tanya Basu, "85-year-old Great-Grandma Scales Mt. Kilimanjaro," *Time*, August 9, 2015, accessed October 14, 2015, http://time.com/3989953/great-grandma-oldest-mt-kilimanjaro/.

3. David Pegg, "25 Oldest People to Accomplish Amazing Feats," List25.com, July 1, 2013, accessed October 14, 2015, http://list25.com/25-oldest-people-to-accomplish-amazing-feats/2/.

4. Pegg, List25.com, accessed October 14, 2015, http://list25.com/25-oldest-people-to-accomplish -amazing-feats/4/.

5. Teng Guo and Lingyi Hu, "Economic Determinants of Happiness: Evidence From the US General Social Survey," Cornell University Library, December 25, 2011, accessed October 14, 2015, http://arxiv.org/abs/1112.5802; Christopher Mims, "Study Suggests Health, Not Wealth, Determines Happiness," ZDNet.com, January 3, 2012, accessed October 14, 2015, http://www.zdnet.com /article/study-suggests-health-not-wealth-determines-happiness/.

6. Mary Shaw, Richard Mitchell, and Danny Dorling, "Time for a Smoke? One Cigarette Reduces Your Life by 11 Minutes," *BMJ* 320.7226 (2000): 53, http://www.ncbi.nlm.nih.gov/pmc/articles /PMC1117323/.

7. J. Lennert Veerman, Genevieve N. Healy, Linda J. Cobiac, et. al., "Television Viewing Time and Reduced Life Expectancy: A Life Table Analysis," *BMJ* 46(2012):927–930. doi:10.1136/bjsports -2011-085662.

8. Steven C. Moore, Alpa V. Patel, Charles E. Matthews, et al., "Leisure Time Physical Activity of Moderate to Vigorous Intensity and Mortality: A Large Pooled Cohort Analysis," *PLOS Medicine* 9(11): e1001335 doi:10.1371/journal.pmed.1001335.

9. "Brisk Daily Walks Can Increase Lifespan, Research Says," *The Guardian*, August 30, 2015, accessed October 14, 2015, http://www.theguardian.com/society/2015/aug/30/brisk-daily-walks -reduce-ageing-increase-life-span-research.

10. "Exercise: 7 Benefits of Regular Physical Activity," Mayo Clinic, accessed October 14, 2015, http://www.mayoclinic.org/healthy-lifestyle/fitness/in-depth/exercise/art-20048389?pg=1.

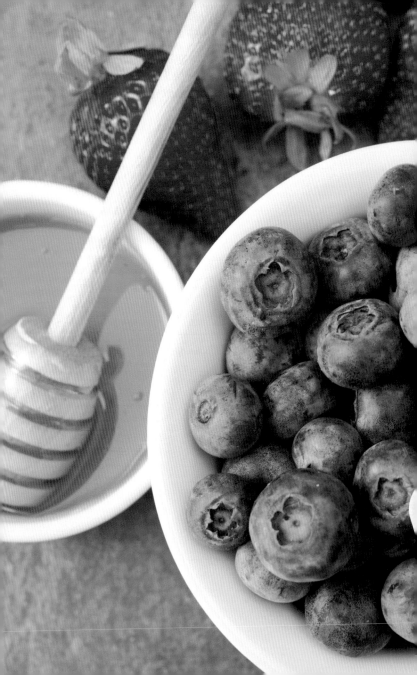

CHAPTER 2

DIET FOR A LIFETIME

Wholesome food strengthens healthy bodies: enjoy it.

Let's suppose you just purchased the car of your dreams: a Porsche Panamera, a Mercedes-Benz S-Class, or an Audi A8. Would you even think of using the lowest grade of fuel possible, neglecting to change the oil, or totally ignoring all of the manufacturer's suggested maintenance checks? Certainly not! If you had just paid more than $90,000 for a luxury car, you would be extremely conscientious about keeping it in optimum condition.

The human body is far more beautiful, complex, and finely tuned than any automobile in the world. Our bodies are a marvel of infinite engineering intelligence. Think of the wonders of a single cell, the complexity of the brain, the intricacies of the heart, or the divine miracle of birth. We stand amazed at the carefully crafted design of the human body. A loving Creator went to infinite lengths to create us, and, like a luxury car, our bodies also need the best possible fuel to power our lives, and that fuel comes from the food we eat. Without premium fuel in a luxury car the mileage goes down, power is lost, and the engine does not run as smoothly. And without the right nutrition, our bodies just do not function properly either.

A balanced diet chosen from the best foods will provide the essential nutrients needed for growth, maintenance, and energy. When we pick low-quality foods or don't eat enough of even the best foods, the body's machinery suffers. And if we overeat highly refined foods, we will lack vital nutrients and can easily become overweight.

Understanding Good Nutrition

We fuel our bodies from the foods we choose to eat. They provide the nutrients essential for a healthy and productive life. Digestion is the intricate process of breaking down food into its individual building blocks so that the body can assimilate and use them to sustain life. This process begins in the mouth, moves to the stomach, then to the small intestines, and finally to the large bowel.

We can divide the nutrients our bodies need into these important categories:

- **Carbohydrates:** In a "premium fuel" diet, the largest portion of carbohydrates should come from rich unrefined sources, such as whole grains, legumes, fruits, and vegetables.
- **Proteins:** Every cell in the body contains proteins. Tissue repair and growth require them. While almost all foods have some protein, animal products such as milk and eggs are also good sources, but not the only ones. Legumes (beans) contain excellent protein.
- **Fats:** These are concentrated sources of energy. We often get too much fat in our diet because we like the flavor it imparts to foods. Many people would rather eat French fries than boiled potatoes. Nuts in moderate amounts provide excellent quality fats, however. The body needs such fats to absorb fat-soluble vitamins.
- **Vitamins:** These are essential organic components of the diet, and are required in small amounts for normal growth and activity. Most occur naturally in various foods. Some are fat-soluble and others water-soluble, and when we do not have a sufficient supply, a deficiency results.
- **Minerals:** These inorganic elements are vital to human health and are easily obtained from both animal and plant foods. Too little of them can lead to a deficiency.
- **Antioxidants and phytochemicals:** Scientists now recognize hundreds of these substances, which protect the body from

disease and some of the effects of aging. We find them primarily in whole grains, fruits, vegetables, and nuts.

You need all these categories of food in order to enjoy good health. The secret is in their combination.

Abundant Nutrition From a Simple Food Plan

What is the best diet for optimum health? A plant-based one. We can easily meet our optimal nutrient needs from the following:

- **Cereals and grains:** These should form the foundation of our diet; they include whole-grain breads, pastas, rice, and corn. When chosen from unrefined (not white) sources, each is rich in dietary fiber, complex carbohydrates, and an array of vitamins and minerals.
- **Fruits and vegetables:** These foods come in a wide variety of colors, flavors, and textures, and are the richest sources of protective phytochemicals, antioxidants, vitamins, and minerals. Many people seem to prefer fruits to vegetables, but we need a balance of both. Foods in this group that are the deepest in color often have the largest amounts of phytochemicals and antioxidants.
- **Legumes, nuts, and seeds:** Legumes, such as beans, peas, and lentils, are an excellent source of good protein, along with minerals, vitamins, and other protective elements. Nuts and seeds provide essential fats, but because they're a concentrated source of calories, we should limit them to no more than one to two servings per day. Nonvegetarians would include fish, fowl, and meat in this group, but these, if consumed at all, should be eaten in moderate amounts only. Some choose to include dairy and eggs in their diets. It is important to recognize that all animal products are high in cholesterol, which may contribute to coronary artery disease. Although animal sources of food provide many important nutrients, including

calcium and vitamin B_{12}, they do pose some health risks. Vitamin B_{12} appears only in animal products and prevents pernicious anemia and neurological disorders, as well as promoting normal cellular division. It's vital for those who choose not to consume any animal products to include sufficient foods fortified with vitamin B_{12} or get it in supplement form on a regular basis.

- **Fats, oils, sweets, and salt:** The body needs such foods only in small amounts.

While the essential fats and sodium are vital for optimum health, excessive amounts can cause serious health problems. Iodine is a necessary trace mineral easily obtained if one uses iodized salt, but it can also be gotten from sea salt, seaweed, or a supplement. We do not require refined sugar for good health, but small amounts add palatability and flavor to food. Nutritional scientists today recognize that plant foods should form the foundation of healthful eating to sustain good health and reduce the risk of disease. One of the most important keys to eating a balanced plant-based diet is selecting a variety of foods whose color, texture, and flavor add interest to the diet. Such foods are best when consumed as they come from nature: not refined or broken down. Whole foods should be the goal.

Today medical science recognizes the advantages of a vegetarian diet. A plant-based vegetarian diet is the following:

- Low in fat, particularly saturated fat
- Low in refined sugar
- Lacking cholesterol (with a total vegetarian diet)
- High in dietary fiber
- High in protective phytochemicals, antioxidants, etc.
- Rich in sources of vitamins and minerals

Having stressed the advantages of adopting certain categories of

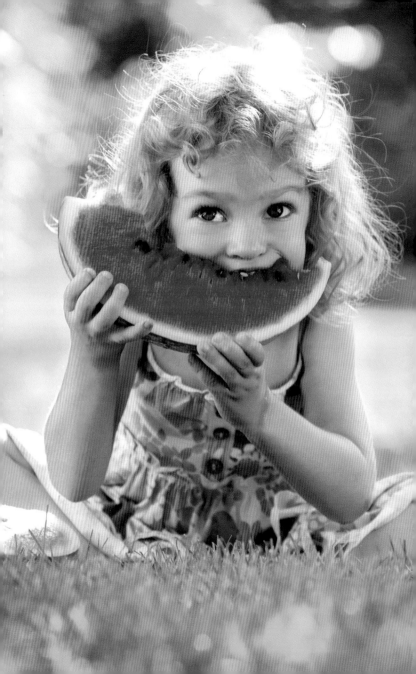

food, especially a vegetarian diet, we now turn our attention to knowing what to take into account when selecting foods.

Principles for Healthful Food Choices

A healthful diet requires good food choices. Keep in mind the following simple principles:

- **Variety:** The most important principle of eating well is selecting a variety of foods. This ensures a wide range of nutrients to support a healthy body, and the various textures, tastes, and colors enhance the pleasure of eating.
- **Quality:** Choose the majority of your food from whole foods, not refined ones. Such foods are nutrient-dense rather than calorie-dense.
- **Moderation**: Some important components of a healthful diet we should eat only in small amounts. Our bodies require adequate amounts of the essential fats as well as small amounts of salt to maintain our electrolytes. But obesity is a growing problem worldwide. It's even possible to eat too much good food! We must balance the amount of energy we consume with the energy we expend in physical activity if we are to remain at a healthful weight.
- **Avoidance**: Highly refined foods that often have large amounts of their nutritional elements removed should be avoided, as should foods and beverages that have no nutritional value (for example, alcohol, coffee, and sodas).

Some people eat as though they don't believe it makes any difference what they consume. But it does. Dr. Gary Fraser, an eminent cardiologist and research scientist, explains how dietary choices and lifestyle affect our longevity and quality of life: "Early in my career as a scientist and physician the great advantages of prevention rather than waiting to treat established disease became clear. Despite the great advances of modern medicine, the expense, sometimes discomfort, and lack of assurance of [a] cure make medical treatment an inferior approach to the control of disease. . . . My colleagues and I have had the opportunity to collect data that in a rigorous scientific fashion allow us to investigate the value of a vegetarian diet. After many years of research by us (and other groups), the evidence is now clear. A plant-based diet provides a host of advantages over a diet containing much meat, as is commonly consumed . . . in the United States and in many other parts of the world."

Dr. Fraser's observation speaks to each one of our desires. Each of us desires "good-quality years." We want to add not only years to our life, but life to our years. That is possible through a change in diet.

CHAPTER 3

ARE YOU AT RISK?

Obesity, which causes several diseases,
need not be devastating: understand it.

Millions of men and women struggle all around the world with noncommunicable diseases: heart conditions, cancers, respiratory diseases, and diabetes. They share four main risk factors: tobacco use, physical inactivity, alcohol, and unhealthy diets. You may be at risk and not fully realize it.

The Obesity Pandemic

The problem of overweight and obesity has become so widespread that health professionals have begun calling it a pandemic. When any disease reaches high levels in a community or geographic area, medical science refers to it as an *epidemic,* but when it occurs in many parts of the world at the same time, it's termed *pandemic.*

According to the World Health Organization, at least 2.8 million people die worldwide each year as a direct result of being overweight or obese. It strikes rich and poor countries alike. Obesity is no longer a characteristic of high-income societies.

You can calculate the amount of overweight or obesity, usually defined as "abnormal or excessive fat accumulation that may impair health," by finding your body mass index (BMI). To do the math, divide your weight in pounds by the square of your height in inches then multiply that answer by 703. If your BMI is equal to or more than 25, you are overweight, and if it is equal to or more than 30, you have obesity. In either case, it is good to start a program of lifestyle changes.

The formula in metric units is: BMI = (weight in kilograms) / (height in meters x height in meters). For example, if you weigh 60 kilograms and are 1.70 meters high, the BMI will be:

BMI = 60 / (1.7 x 1.7) = 20.8 (you are in the normal category).

If you do not want to bother to make the calculations, just go to the Internet for a BMI calculator. You will find many, both in English and metric units.[1]

What does your BMI say? Are you at risk? Are you overweight? Is your blood pressure normal? Do you eat large servings of fatty, high-calorie, refined, and processed foods? Does your diet come mainly from fast-food outlets? If so, you're headed for trouble, or you may already have problems with your health and not be aware of it.

The media advertises many "miraculous" plans for losing weight, but the best and safest is a radical change in lifestyle as proposed in this book.

Obesity + Diabetes = "Diabesity"

Several health problems result from obesity, including increased risk of heart disease, high blood pressure, and certain cancers. Yet one of the more common is diabetes, which we will focus on here. More than one-third of a billion people in the world have diabetes—about one of every 20 people on earth! The countries with the largest likely diabetes increase by 2030 include China, India, and the United States. They all lead many others, both rich and poor.[2] Obesity, defined as a person weighing 20 percent or more above the normal weight for their height, is the number one risk factor for developing type 2 diabetes. As many as 80 percent of people with type 2 diabetes are obese. The two conditions of diabetes and obesity are so closely linked that many health experts refer to them as one disease, which they have dubbed *diabesity*.

The rate of diabetes has risen dramatically in the general popula-tion in recent years, as has the incidence of obesity, the number one risk factor for diabetes. An estimated 3.4 million people worldwide die from the complications of diabetes each year. The World Health

Organization projects that diabetes will be the seventh-leading cause of death by the year 2030.[3] If diabetes is such a mortal enemy, then it is important to know how to overcome it.

What Is Diabetes?

Running through our bodies is an intricate system of blood vessels that we can think of as pipes ranging in size from about one inch (2.5 centimeters) to as small as .0002 inches, just enough room for one red blood cell to squeeze through at a time. The blood carries all the nutrients needed by every cell in your body to perform their correct functions. The energy source for cells is a simple form of sugar called *glucose*. Too much glucose (sugar) can damage the cells. The body, therefore, has an amazing way of regulating the amount of sugar in the blood. It does so by *insulin,* a substance produced by cells in the pancreas.

Diabetes is a chronic disease in which the amount of sugar carried in the blood does not get regulated as it should be. Either the body does not produce insulin normally (type 1 diabetes, also known as T1DM), or it develops resistance to insulin, which means the sugar is not effectively controlled (type 2 diabetes, or T2DM).

A third type of diabetes can develop in pregnant women who have not had diabetes before. It most often occurs after three months of pregnancy. Obesity in pregnancy is a leading risk factor for childhood obesity. It also increases the potential for high blood pressure during pregnancy, as well as other severe complications of pregnancy. Babies born to obese mothers are more likely to have birth defects and heart problems.[4]

Diabesity during pregnancy can lead to significant complications for both mother and child. High maternal blood glucose damages the delicate functioning of the baby's cells, which leads to cell death and increased abnormalities in the child.

People who have diabetes often complain of passing markedly increased amounts of urine. The high levels of sugar in the blood spill over into the urine. The increased fluid (and sugar) loss through urine stimulates the thirst mechanism, causing them to drink a lot of water

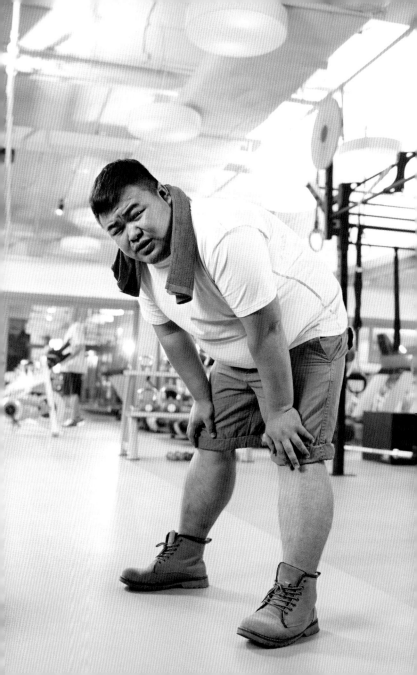

to compensate. Body weight may decrease, and long-term damage to nerves and blood vessels (the latter injury can lead to heart attack, stroke, and kidney failure) may result. The destruction of neglected blood vessels can cause gangrene of the limbs.

Prevention, Reversal, or Control of Diabetes

Careful blood sugar control helps prevent the negative effects of diabesity and improves pregnancy outcomes, but it can be difficult to achieve. A diet low in refined carbohydrates and saturated fat, combined with moderate exercise, can improve the health of the mother and baby, because such lifestyle changes help control weight during pregnancy. For women who are morbidly (very) obese and contemplating pregnancy, surgical interventions can be helpful alternatives to diet and exercise to regulate weight and prevent onset of, or reverse, diabetes. Through rigorous monitoring and strict adherence to health plans, it *is* possible to avert diabesity and its complications.

Diabetics must carefully control their blood sugar levels and sometimes may require insulin (injections)—most commonly in type 1 diabetes. Some patients with type 2 diabetes require sugar-lowering tablets, but the mainstay of treatment is changing to a plant-based diet rich in fresh fruit, fresh vegetables, and nuts, and low in refined carbohydrates and saturated fats. Lifestyle changes such as exercise and weight loss can prevent or delay the onset of type 2 diabetes.

The American Diabetes Association discussed the value of a plant-based diet and made this observation: "A vegetarian diet is a healthy option, even if you have diabetes. Research supports that following this type of diet can help prevent and manage diabetes. . . . Vegan diets [a total plant-based diet] are naturally higher in fiber, much lower in saturated fat, and cholesterol-free when compared to a traditional American diet. . . . The high fiber in this diet may help you feel full for a longer time after eating and may help you eat less over time. . . . This diet also tends to cost less. Meat, poultry, and fish are usually the most expensive foods we eat."[5]

Such lifestyle measures bring huge benefits and are not too expensive. While they demand commitment and time, they do help to keep the blood glucose close to normal and prevent damage to the eyes, kidneys, and blood vessels—especially of the lower limbs. British physician and researcher Denis Burkitt was right when he commented, "If people are constantly falling off a cliff, you could place ambulances under the cliff or build a fence on the top of the cliff. We are placing all too many ambulances under the cliff."

Many people are essentially saying, "Doc, let me live like I want, eat what I want, smoke and drink what I want, then give me a magic pill to keep me well." But there is a much better way than disregarding the laws of health and hoping beyond hope to stay well. Instead, we can build "fences" to protect ourselves and our children against premature disease and death by eating a healthy natural diet, exercising regularly, getting adequate rest, drinking plenty of water, developing positive relationships, and having faith in a God who really cares for us. We have an enormous challenge and also a great opportunity. Prevention is preferable to an ambulance. It is not only better than the cure—it *is* the cure. As adults, we have the privilege of modeling healthful behaviors for our children that will protect them from the raging pandemic.

At the same time, our own health will benefit. We need to be physically active and encourage our children to exercise too. We must be responsible architects of their choices, providing the most healthful food options as priorities in our budgets. That applies especially to pregnant mothers, who shape both their children's choices and their own future health, or possible lack thereof.

The Bible has great advice and encouragement for guiding our children's, as well as our own, decisions in health and general behaviors: "Start children off on the way they should go, and even when they are old they will not turn from it" (Proverbs 22:6, NIV). We see the importance of repetition in instruction and example well described in the following advice regarding God's law and directions: "These commandments that I give you today are to be on your hearts. Impress them on your children. Talk about them when you sit at home and when you walk along the road, when you lie down and when you get up" (Deuteronomy 6:6, 7, NIV). As parents we need to invest time, love, example, and perseverance from conception of the baby until the child becomes independent of parental care.

Scripture reminds us that we are "fearfully and wonderfully made" (Psalm 139:14). Our response of praise and gratitude, therefore, should be to honor our Creator in all things: "Whether you eat or drink or whatever you do, do it all for the glory of God" (1 Corinthians 10:31, NIV). He is faithful in helping to guide our decisions and choices from portion sizes and the foods best suited to our needs, to exercise and adequate rest. One of the greatest motivations to keep our bodies in good health is to honor the God who created us. There is something much more than merely being healthy for health's sake, as important as that is, or a personal desire to live longer on earth. Even if we meticulously follow the laws of health, all of us will die sometime unless our Lord returns first. Our bodies are not a fun house. They are the temples of the Holy Spirit, and that makes all the difference.

A number of years ago Dr. Albert Reece, dean of the School of Medicine at the University of Maryland, was helping a woman who had smoked for decades to quit. He tried everything, but she just could not seem to stop. She might be off cigarettes for a few days, but then would start smoking again. One day Dr. Reece, who is a Christian, shared the fact that her body was the temple of the Holy Spirit and that Jesus through the Holy Spirit longed to dwell in her body. He explained that the choices she made in caring for her body would determine in part her fitness for eternity. A week or so later, when he visited her to offer encouragement, she said, "I quit. I have not smoked since our last visit. When I wanted to take a puff, I pictured the Holy Spirit choking. I no longer desire to defile my body temple with tobacco. I want to present my body to Jesus in the best possible condition when He returns."

Would you like to offer your body as a living sacrifice to Jesus as

His temple for His Holy Spirit to dwell in? Why don't you invite Him right now to strengthen your resolve and commitment to healthful living? He will immediately come to your aid. If you need a change of heart by the Great Physician, God can do it, as the Bible says in Ezekiel 36:26: "I will give you a new heart and put a new spirit in you. . . . I will move you to follow my decrees and be careful to keep my laws" (NIV). We all need help to make changes in our behavior. Look for help outside of yourself—seek God's help. You cannot do it without Him, but He will not do it without your choice and cooperation. Ask a close friend or family member to partner with you and encourage accountability and pray together. You'll be glad you did as you experience positive results and live life to the full!

---

1. For example, "Calculate Your Body Mass Index," National Heart, Lung, and Blood Institute, www.nhlbi.nih.gov/guidelines/obesity/BMI/bmicalc.htm.

2. S. Wild, G. Roglic, A. Green, R. Sicree, and H. King, "Global Prevalence of Diabetes: Estimates for the Year 2000 and Projections for 2030," *Diabetes Care* 27 (2004): 1047–1053.

3. World Health Organization, "Fact Sheet No. 312," available at www.who.int/mediacentre/factsheets/fs312/en/.

4. K. J. Stothard et al., "Maternal Overweight and Obesity and the Risk of Congenital Anomalies: A Systematic Review and Meta-analysis," *Journal of the American Medical Association* 301 (2009): 636–650.

5. Available at www.diabetes.org/food-and-fitness/food/planning-meals/meal-planning-for-vegetarians/.

CHAPTER 4

FIT FOR LIFE

Exercise is a choice: practice it.

M ost things that are worthwhile take effort, and that is especially true of our health. Good health is not something that comes by some stroke of luck. It is not a matter of chance. Although each one of us has a different genetic makeup and predisposition to disease, following the principles of health that our Creator has written on every nerve and tissue of our bodies contributes to our overall well-being. When you have worked all day and are just about worn out, it takes real discipline to exercise. Or when you are tired and would much rather munch on peanuts while watching your favorite comedy on television, it takes a determined choice to get off the couch and exercise. Your goal is to evaluate where you are, consult with your health-care provider, and begin regular, systematic exercise appropriate for your age and abilities. For some younger people it may be more vigorous than for those of us who are a little older.

What will it take to motivate you to begin and maintain a regular exercise program? If you aren't regularly exercising now, what will it require to get you going?

Exercise Essentials

Exercise is one way to start your body moving in the direction of good health. The father of medicine, Hippocrates, once said, "If we could give every individual the right amount of nourishment and exercise, not too little and not too much, we would have found the safest way to health." That is also our challenge in the twenty-first century. Most of us stare at one screen after another—smartphones, iPads, e-readers, and computers—up to eight hours a day. Then, if you add TV watching, we end up spending more time in front of screens than we do sleeping! With continued mechanization, even manual occupations require less physical activity. Vibrant health requires activity, movement, and exercise. Good health isn't only about not being ill—it's about being happy and feeling whole from a physical, mental, social, and spiritual point of view. Exercise and activity help to make those outcomes a reality.

Above all, exercise is a part of the total health package. Ellen White, an inspired health educator, outlined a balanced, multifaceted approach to healthful living that has stood the test of time and science: "Pure air, sunlight, abstemiousness, rest, exercise, proper diet, the use of water, trust in divine power—these are the true remedies. Every person should have a knowledge of nature's remedial agencies and how to apply them."[1]

The goal of exercise is to maintain or enhance our overall physical fitness and general health. People exercise to strengthen muscles, optimize the cardiovascular system, control body weight, develop athletic skills, improve physical appearance, facilitate general wellness and mental alertness, and also to socialize and have fun. It is the single most important thing we can do to enhance our longevity.

Ellen White offers another helpful perspective. "The body is the only medium through which the mind and the soul are developed for the up building of character."[2] In the same way that a good foundation is the basis of a building structure, a well-functioning body facilitates the development of one's mental capabilities and, ultimately, one's character.

Benefits of Exercise

Unless you overexercise or exercise in the wrong manner, physical activity is always beneficial. It's never too late to start, and some exercise is better than none at all.

Exercise facilitates sustainable weight loss and improves posture and appearance. It also reduces the risk and the progression of heart disease, diabetes, cancer, and Alzheimer's, as well as premature death. Have you ever felt stiff and wished you had more flexibility? Exercise increases body flexibility, strengthens bones and joints, protects against fractures, and builds healthy muscles. The benefits that follow exercise include lowered blood pressure, lowered heart rate, and a decreased risk for both obesity and diabetes. If you feel too tired to exercise, remember that exercise increases energy, vitality, speed, and performance. Fitness facilitates recovery from injury and illness.

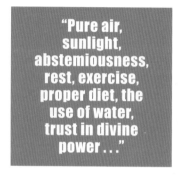

"Pure air, sunlight, abstemiousness, rest, exercise, proper diet, the use of water, trust in divine power . . ."

Now that we have considered the physical benefits of exercise, what about its mental benefits? If ever there existed a magic formula for health, it is exercise. A good walk in the park or jog around the block improves learning, retention, and overall mental function. It is a great stress reliever and enhances overall psychological health. The rates of depression decrease, and self-esteem increases in those who exercise. Have you ever noticed that when you have exercised, you sleep better that night?

Exercise also provides some surprising social benefits. It facilitates emotional intelligence and conflict resolution, strengthens intimacy and sexual life, and promotes feelings of happiness. Since exercise increases the flow of oxygen carrying blood cells to the brain, it also enhances our ability to meditate, pray, and study the Bible. Systematic exercise increases our capacity to appreciate spiritual things. With the renewed energy that comes from exercise we will also have a greater desire to serve others.

A Plan and Pointers

One of the world's leading professional organizations in exercise physiology, the American College of Sports Medicine, has designed a template

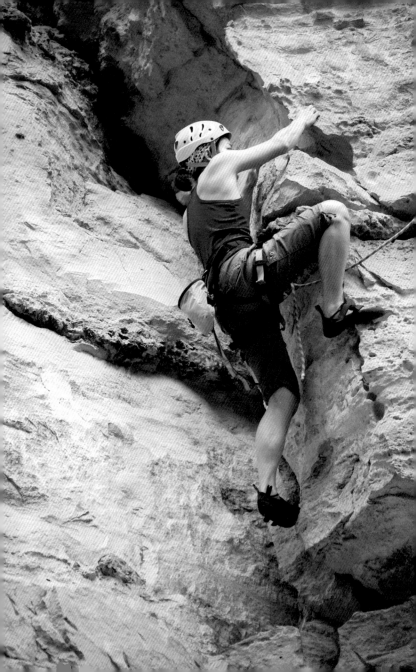

for a healthy amount of exercise. We each need at least 150 minutes of moderate exercise per week. For most, this is a very reachable goal. All that we need is a sidewalk, a trail in the woods, a treadmill—and a small time commitment that adds up to fewer than three hours a week, or about 30 minutes a day, for exercise. Surprisingly enough, you do not need to be a world-class sprinter or weight lifter to get enough exercise. A brisk walk for a minimum of 30 minutes five times a week will do. Recent research indicates that we do not need to take the exercise all at one time. Three 10-minute sessions will give the same benefits that 30 minutes will confer.

Of course, it's not enough just to read and talk about exercise—you must do it! Someone has said, "All the talking about walking will not take the place of a good walk." Review your past habits, assess what they are now, and decide what you want them to be. Don't worry about whether you'll be successful or not. Simply determine to do your best from this point forward. Then start.

1. Plan: While there are many exercise programs available, here are four principles to keep in mind: the frequency and intensity of your exercise program, along with the time and type of your exercise regime. But always consult with your physician before starting it. Let's look briefly at each of the four components of a good exercise program.

- **Frequency** has to do with how often you exercise. For cardio exercise, most exercise specialists suggest moderate exercise five days a week or intense cardio three days a week to improve your health. For weight loss, you may need to do up to six or more days a week. And for strength training, the recommended frequency is two or three nonconsecutive days a week with at least a one- or two-day break between sessions.
- **Intensity** involves how hard you exercise. The general rule for cardio exercise is to work in your target heart-rate zone and focus on a variety of intensities to stimulate different energy systems. For strength training, the exercises you do, the amount

of weight you lift, and your sets and repetitions determine the intensity of your workouts.

- **Time** concerns how long you should exercise. Exercise guidelines suggest that your goal should be 30–60 minutes per session. That does not mean you will start by exercising for an hour. It may take you some time to work your way up to that level of cardio exercise. Begin slowly. If you have not been exercising for a while, you cannot make up for 10 years of lack of it in one day. Its intensity and your fitness level will determine the duration of your exercise. The harder you work, the shorter your workouts will be.

- For cardio exercise you can do any **type** of activity that increases your heart rate, such as running, walking, cycling, swimming, sports, etc. Strength training includes basically any exercise with which you're using some form of resistance (bands, dumbbells, machines, etc.) to work your muscles.

Remember these four principles:

a. **Frequency:** exercise regularly.
b. **Intensity:** exercise strenuously.
c. **Time:** exercise at least 30 minutes a day.
d. **Type:** incorporate both aerobic exercise and strength-building exercise into your exercise program.

As you follow this basic exercise outline, it will help you to adjust your workouts to avoid boredom, overuse injuries, and weight-loss plateaus.

The simplest measure of adequate aerobic exercise is to obtain a pedometer (step counter) and walk the recommended 10,000 steps per day every day! This will ensure basic personal fitness.

2. Pointers: In order for your program to work regardless of whether you're a beginner or a "pro," here are some helpful pointers.

- Move. Nothing will happen unless you take action. Just do it!
- Use the three-step change model. First, know where you are now; second, decide where you want to be; third, develop a plan to get there.
- Learn more about exercises. Begin to research subjects related to your particular interests. Emphasize the positive aspects of practicing a healthful lifestyle—think it, believe it, talk it. Start and restart with the belief that you will be successful.
- Evaluate your performance. Some people find it helpful to keep a log of when they start exercising, then make notes of their progress (you will find many good exercise logs available on the Internet to assist you).
- Get moving. Start today and don't stop. Continuity is essential. Remember that the three major exercise stoppers are: (a) procrastination, (b) lack of persistence, and (c) self-defeating attitudes. You may not achieve all of your goals, but do not become discouraged. Never give up on your exercise.

Remember that all the good you do for your body will only complement and support your spiritual and mental objectives. Exercise, and relish the positive feelings that it brings. Evaluate your progress and remain motivated.

Extra Strength

Good religion is complemented by good health habits, which, of necessity, should include exercise. The body and soul are wedded to each other, and it's proper to pray that they both may prosper to the glory of God. "Beloved, I pray that you may prosper in all things and be in health, just as your soul prospers" (3 John 2, NKJV). Whenever we face problems, obstacles, or challenges in doing God's will, including exercising, we have the privilege of asking Him for help to strengthen our resolve. As we choose to live in harmony with the principles of positive, healthful living, He will strengthen us to do the right thing. We're not in this battle alone. You can do all things through Christ, who strengthens you (see Philippians 4:13).

Your body is the temple of God, through which He communicates. Exercise helps to keep that temple in good shape so that you can perceive what God wants you to do, and then be able to do it. Many people overeat, have bad habits, and don't exercise. Then they pray that God may heal their bodies. Isn't it rather presumptuous of us to think that we can knowingly violate the laws of health and expect God to give us good health? Although exercise will not guarantee good health, not exercising may very well guarantee we will not have it.

Each day, plan to spend some time in exercise. Use this time to breathe a prayer and fellowship with your Maker. It will invigorate your mind, body, and spirit. With exercising and good health there's no room for excuses and procrastination. We have to make it happen to maintain health and wellness. No one can do it for you but you. Now it's up to you!

---

1. Ellen G. White, *Counsels on Health* (Mountain View, Calif.: Pacific Press Pub. Assn., 1923), 90.
2. Ellen G. White, *My Life Today* (Washington, D.C.: Review and Herald Pub. Assn., 1952), 78.

CHAPTER 5

INVIGORATED BY AIR, WATER, AND SUNSHINE

The environment energizes: enjoy it, but don't destroy it.

The rush of air that passed their faces was invigorating! It didn't matter that the temperature was near freezing. Orville was guiding the first controlled flight, and his brother Wilbur was running alongside the wing of the flying machine. On December 17, 1903, the Wright brothers made a total of four short, but historic, flights. The success of this great achievement made the preparation and practice worthwhile! The amazing characteristics of air, including lift, make flight possible. Other properties of air allow living creatures to breathe and exist, and often rekindle the joy of life following an invigorating after-breakfast run, bike ride, or tour in the beauty of nature surrounded by air and water and bathed in sunshine!

Air—the Breath of Life

Atmospheric air comprises a mixture of gases: 20.95 percent oxygen (O_2), 0.04 percent carbon dioxide (CO_2), 78.09 percent nitrogen (N_2), and the balance of inert substances such as argon and helium. Oxygen is the vital and life-sustaining component of air. Breathing is the process that moves the air in and out of the lungs and sustains the cycle of taking in oxygen and releasing carbon dioxide. This process allows for the exchange of the breathtaking amount of 20,000 liters (more than 5,000 gallons) of air per day into and out of the body![1] Of this, approximately two quarts of oxygen are carried through the lungs, blood, and other tissues at any given time. Oxygen enters the blood from the lungs by a process called *diffusion*. The heart and circulatory system then pump this life-giving blood to every tissue of the body, supplying oxygen to all tissues and cells. The cells need oxygen for their efficient function and metabolism.

The body has delicate and intricate mechanisms to maintain normal oxygen levels. The coordinating control center is in the brain stem; and it measures the levels of oxygen and carbon dioxide in the blood, to regulate the rate and depth of breathing. You cannot hold your breath for long periods: as the carbon dioxide levels increase, an unstoppable "air hunger" develops, forcing you to breathe. This is an amazing and miraculous reflex, which is lifesaving. If your breathing stops, the body's oxygen levels drop dangerously low within minutes, and brain damage and ultimately death ensue. Brain cells begin to die within five minutes of being deprived of oxygen, emphasizing the truth of the American Lung Association's former motto: "It's a matter of life and breath."

During exercise, your demand for oxygen increases and more carbon dioxide is produced. Reflex mechanisms are activated in the brain, and your breathing becomes deeper and more rapid. During periods of rest, your rate of breathing is lower because your carbon dioxide production is lower. Your amazing body has been designed to maintain just the right amount of oxygen for its needs at any given moment.

Apart from sustaining human life, the earth's air has many protective qualities. On a global scale, the air and its suspended water vapor protect the world and its inhabitants from solar radiation and the cold vacuum of outer space. The air assists with the recycling of water and helps to moderate the climate. It provides an atmospheric envelope, sustaining life with varied needs for oxygen. To enjoy optimal health, humans need fresh, clean air.

In some places, the air is often polluted. This may occur through inadequate ventilation of dwellings, especially where open fires are used for cooking and heating. In cities, the air in buildings is often recirculated through air-conditioning systems and may increase the pollution both indoors and outdoors. City smog, tobacco smoke, and industrial pollutants are additional culprits.

Fresh, clean air can usually be found in abundance in natural outdoor environments, especially around trees, which have been called the "lungs of the earth." It is present also in the vicinity of green plants, mountains, and forests, and near moving water such as lakes, oceans, waterfalls, and rivers, and after a rainfall. The air, when unpolluted, is invigorating. Deep breathing of fresh air imparts an improved sense of well-being. It increases the rate and quality of growth in plants and animals and improves the protective mechanisms of the lungs.

The air around us may be laden with air pollutants, especially on freeways, near airports, and in industrialized areas. Polluted, smoke-filled air has been associated with increased anxiety, migraine headaches, nausea, vomiting, eye discomfort and dryness, and respiratory congestion. The World Health Organization estimates that more than 2 million people die every year from breathing in tiny pollutant particles present in indoor and outdoor pollution.[2] Some 6 million people—mostly children—die each year from acute respiratory infections, complicated particularly by indoor pollution often originating from unvented or poorly vented cooking facilities. Breathing polluted air may contribute to heart disease,[3] stroke,[4] lung cancer, bronchitis, and other lung infections. Research has shown that being exposed to air pollution for long periods of time can speed up the cognitive decline in older women and increase the progression of dementia.[5]

A very preventable form of air pollution and significant danger to innocent bystanders comes from secondhand tobacco smoke. In homes where parents and other family members smoke, children and spouses are often the victims of secondhand smoke (SHS). These children suffer more lower respiratory and middle-ear infections.[6] Exposure to SHS increases the number and severity of asthma episodes in asthmatic children.[7] There is evidence linking tobacco smoke to sudden infant death syndrome.[8] Adults exposed to SHS have an increased risk of lung cancer—24 percent in women and 30 percent in men living with smokers.[9] Nonsmokers exposed to SHS in the workplace have a 16 to 19 percent increased risk of developing lung cancer.[10]

How can you ensure that you get adequate amounts of clean air and vital oxygen?

- Avoid tobacco smoke—both SHS and firsthand smoke. Don't start smoking!
- Take deep breaths, and exercise regularly. Avoid shallow breathing, and ensure that the lungs are expanded fully.
- Take intentional breaks during work and leisure time to breathe deeply—outdoors if this is safe and feasible.
- Pay attention to your posture: stand and sit up straight, with your shoulders back, and breathe deeply.
- Seek help to assist you to stop smoking. Even electronic cigarettes have proven to be health hazards.

In short, nurture your brain's function! The cells most sensitive to a lack of oxygen are those of the brain, which is the seat of judgment, reason, intellect, and the will. It is the control center of your entire being. Ensure that you breathe healthful, fresh air, and become invigorated in your body, mind, and spirit!

Water—the Liquid of Life

Next to air, water is the most vital element needed for both survival and quality of life. Just a quick analysis of the human body reveals the importance of water in the body's makeup and function. By weight, a newborn infant is approximately 75 percent water and an adult about 60 to 70 percent. The gray matter of the brain (the area where thought, planning, cognition, and intelligence reside) is approximately 85 percent water. Not surprisingly, blood is 83 percent water, and even hard tissue such as bone is 20 to 25 percent water.[11] Almost every cell and tissue of the body not only contain water but are bathed in water and need water for their efficient functioning.

Water can truly be described as the liquid of life! It is all of the

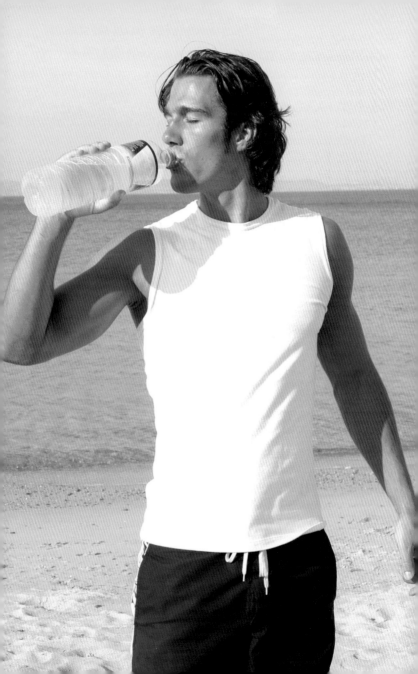

following:

- The transport system within the body
- The lubricant for movement
- A facilitator of digestion
- The prime transporter of waste via the kidneys
- Important in regulating body temperature
- The major constituent of circulating blood

About two-thirds of our daily water requirements come from ingested liquid and about one-third from our food (a very small amount of water is formed in the process of normal metabolism). Fruits and vegetables have a higher water content than other food groups. Just as with air and breathing, the body has the most intricate, efficient, and brilliantly designed mechanisms to maintain the water and electrolyte balance. This process ensures that the internal "environment" of every cell and function remains optimal, with adequate hydration.

What happens when our fluid intake is inadequate? The body cuts back on fluid loss by decreasing the amount of sweat and urine produced. Even these efficient compensatory mechanisms may be overcome if an insufficient fluid intake persists. Dehydration follows with the impairment of temperature control, the retention of toxic waste products, and the thickening and possible "sludging" of the blood flow, which increases the possibility of blood clots forming. This may, in turn, cause heart attacks or strokes. Other symptoms or problems related to dehydration may include the following:

- Dizziness
- Headache
- Kidney stones
- Gallstones[12]
- Constipation[13]

The adequate intake of water, ensuring optimal hydration, could solve many common symptoms and health problems from headaches to constipation in all age groups. The very young and the elderly are particularly at risk. In 1995, it was estimated that the adequate hydration of older people could save thousands of days of hospitalization and millions of dollars each year.[14] Better hydration across all age groups could lead to improved health globally, especially if water sources are safe, clean, and secure. However, there may be an associated decrease in the profits of the laxative industry, which is a multibillion dollar operation in the United States alone!

You may ask, How much water should I be drinking each day? The amount of water needed varies according to your activities and local weather conditions. The more active you are the more you perspire to maintain a normal body temperature, and therefore the more water you need to drink to keep up with the losses. As the ambient temperature increases, the need for additional water intake increases.

A practical and easy way to assess whether you are drinking enough water is to ensure that your urine is pale and approaches the color of water. In this way, you can be confident of maintaining adequate hydration. It is important to know that some medication, such as antibiotics (especially antituberculosis treatment), and even some vitamin supplements may impart a darker yellow or an orange color to the urine. Otherwise, this color test is a practical and useful guide.

Here are some practical tips:

- Begin the day with 1 to 2 glasses of water, because the body becomes less hydrated overnight through the "invisible" (imperceptible) water loss from breathing and perspiration.
- Continue to drink water at regular intervals throughout the day.
- When exercising or when in hot climates or environments, drink enough water to quench your thirst, *plus* an additional third of that required volume (e.g., 1 liter to quench your

thirst after a strenuous workout plus 300 milliliters would mean that the adequate replacement amount would be a total of 1.3 liters).

• Drink water that is pure and clean. It is the healthiest drink available and most suited to the body's needs.

One day while seated in a restaurant in Geneva, a waiter asked me what I wanted to drink. I automatically responded, "Do you have anything sugar-free?" He straightened his already-upright posture even further, purposefully focused on me, and bluntly blurted, "Yes. We have water!" I was initially annoyed at his reply, but it served me well; for years now, I have seldom chosen anything else. Water has no calories, few electrolytes, and is physiologically friendly. Yes. We have water. Let's drink it heartily!

In addition, water is a cleansing agent, within and without. Regular bathing keeps the body clean and hygienic. Frequent hand-washing with soap and water may reduce the transmission of many infectious agents, especially influenza, the common cold, and infectious diarrhea. Water is a wonderful, natural agent, with many healthful and preventive properties—and it's there for the using!

Sunshine—a Provider of Energy

What complements the refreshing feeling of a breeze in one's face following a rain shower? Warm, welcoming, and comforting rays of sunshine! Sunshine adds sparkle to water and changes the hues of the sky depending on the time of day. It gives light, not only so we may see but also to aid our metabolism of calcium by producing vitamin D precursors in the skin. Placing all of these natural health-promoting agents together—air, water, and sunshine—one might think that the environment was planned with humankind in mind. It's as if we were expected. We are wonderfully designed and created, as is the world we inhabit.

The sun is central to the provision of energy for our planet. Much of its radiation promotes health and well-being. It is essential for the growth of plants, vegetation, and photosynthesis in plant life—the food-production mechanism. This, in turn, impacts the lives of all who eat those plants. Sunlight powers the recycling of water through its evaporation into the clouds and its distillation as rain.

Sunshine converts *cholecalciferol,* the precursor of vitamin D, into active vitamin D. Vitamin D helps to ensure the maintenance and repairing of our bones, but it has also been found to have many other important bodily functions. Many people lose out on these benefits because of working long hours indoors and having insufficient exposure to the sun.

Darkly pigmented skin does not permit the ultraviolet rays of the sun to work efficiently in the production of vitamin D, resulting in lower levels. People who live in the extreme northern or southern parts of the world also have difficulties obtaining enough vitamin D, due to less sun exposure during certain times of the year.

There is an important caution regarding sunlight exposure: dermatologists have noted and shown a causal relationship between sunburn and skin cancer, especially when there is excessive exposure in childhood. It is important to use appropriate sunscreen protection; however, this does decrease vitamin D production. Paradoxically, vitamin D is thought to be an important factor in controlling the growth of other cancers, such as prostate cancer. Sunlight exposure is, therefore, important to health.[15] The safest times to benefit from sunshine are before 10 A.M. and after 4 P.M. Exposure without sunscreen should be limited to 20 minutes.

Sunshine kills certain bacteria, so let it stream into your home. Glass gives some skin protection by blocking UV rays. Sunlight exposure stimulates the production of other hormones, such as melatonin, which assists our sleep, and serotonin, which affects our mood. Our "external" environment influences our "internal" environment, and we see this with the three natural health promoters: sunshine, air, and water. Seasonal affective disorder—first described in 1984 by Dr.

Norman Rosenthal, then a psychiatrist at the National Institute of Mental Health—affects many during the winter months, when the shorter days limit one's sunshine exposure. This can lead to a loss of energy, an alteration in the appetite, sleepiness during the day, irritability, and depression.[16] Individuals with this problem benefit from exposure to bright light.

A very important warning: do not attempt to substitute sunshine exposure with a tanning bed. Tanning beds have been shown to be associated with an aggressive and relentless skin cancer called *melanoma*. In your quest to use natural health promoters, use the real thing.

We are surrounded by an environment filled with breathtaking beauty but also healing and health-promoting properties. Air, water, and sunlight affect not only our physical health but our mental, emotional, and—as we contemplate the gift of life and health—our spiritual health as well.

We all seek wholeness, the filling of the sometimes existent "emptiness" in facets of our lives. Some have termed this the "God-shaped space." Our interactions with one other, our environment, and the health-promoting blessings of air, water, and sunshine give us pause to think. We have the privilege and responsibility to ensure we breathe the freshest air; drink pure, clean water; and wisely benefit from the warmth and light of sunshine. We should also care for this beautiful environment and not pollute it!

But we cannot do this alone. We need the sustaining power and grace of the loving Creator God.

"In the matchless gift of His Son, God has encircled the whole world with an atmosphere of grace as real as the air which circulates around the globe. All who choose to breathe this life-giving atmosphere will live and grow up to the stature of men and women in Christ Jesus."[17]

As we choose and enjoy the vital and fulfilled life, we need to breathe deeply, use pure water, enjoy the sunshine wisely, and never forget the indwelling presence of God, the Water and Breath of Life.

1. "Anatomy of the Lungs," Cedars-Sinai, accessed June 18, 2015, www.cedars-sinai.edu/Patients/Programs-and-Services/Lung-Institute/Patient-Guide/Anatomy-of-the-Lungs/.

2. World Health Organization, "Tackling the Global Clean Air Challenge," press release, September 26, 2011, http://bit.ly/p90Y2g.

3. R. Bhatia, "Policy and Regulatory Action Can Reduce Harms From Particulate Pollution," *Archives of Internal Medicine* 172, no. 3 (2012): 227, 228.

4. G. A. Wellenius et al., "Ambient Air Pollution and the Risk of Ischemic Stroke," *Archives of Internal Medicine* 172, no. 3 (2012): 229–234, doi:10.1001/archinternmed.2011.732.

5. J. Weuve et al., "Exposure to Particulate Air Pollution and Cognitive Decline in Older Women," *Archives of Internal Medicine* 172, no. 3 (2012): 219–227.

6. D. P. Strachan and D. G. Cook, "Health Effects of Passive Smoking. 1. Parental Smoking and Lower Respiratory Illness in Infancy and Early Childhood," *Thorax* 52, no. 10 (1997): 905–914.

7. D. P. Strachan and D. G. Cook, "Health Effects of Passive Smoking. 3. Parental Smoking and Prevalence of Respiratory Symptoms and Asthma in School Age Children," *Thorax* 52, no. 12 (1997): 1081–1094.

8. "About Second Hand Smoke," World Health Organization, accessed June 29, 2015, http://www.who.int/tobacco/research/secondhand_smoke/about/en/.

9. A. K. Hackshaw, M. R. Law, and N. J. Wald, "The Accumulated Evidence on Lung Cancer and Environmental Tobacco Smoke," *British Medical Journal* 315 (1997): 980–988.

10. "Frequently Asked Questions About Second Hand Smoke," World Health Organization, accessed June 29, 2015, http://www.who.int/tobacco/research/secondhand_smoke/faq/en/.

11. M. G. Hardinge, *A Philosophy of Health* (Loma Linda, Calif.: Loma Linda University School of Public Health, 1980), 37.

12. E. Braunwald et al., eds., *Harrison's Principles of Internal Medicine,* 17th ed. (New York: McGraw-Hill, 2011), 1616, 1617.

13. "The Basics of Constipation," WebMD, accessed April 4, 2012, www.webmd.com/digestive-disorders/digestive-diseases-constipation#causes.

14. A. D. Weinberg and K. L. Minaker, "Dehydration: Evaluation and Management in Older Adults, Council on Scientific Affairs, American Medical Association," *Journal of the American Medical Association* 274, no. 19 (November 1995): 1552–1556.

15. H. G. Ainsleigh, "Beneficial Effects of Sun Exposure on Cancer Mortality," *American Journal of Preventive Medicine* 22, no. 1 (January 1993): 132–140.

16. D. L. Kasper et al., eds., *Harrison's Principles of Internal Medicine,* 19th ed. (New York: McGraw-Hill, 2015), 2715.

17. Ellen G. White, *Steps to Christ* (Mountain View, Calif.: Pacific Press® Publishing Association, 1956), 68.

CHAPTER 6

HEALTHY RELATIONSHIPS

Love matters: invest in it.

Research has shown that supportive relationships strengthen the immune system and increase our ability to fight off illness and disease. One such study indicated that just three weekly visits by relatives and close friends improved the immune function in the seniors.[1] The other side of the coin is also true. Scientific investigation has documented that abusive relationships may damage our health. Exposure to physical, sexual, or emotional violence, or the ongoing stress related to abuse, has links to many health problems. Adverse childhood experiences appear to produce several physical health problems later in adulthood. The traumatic childhood events include "verbal, physical, or sexual abuse, as well as family dysfunction," such as witnessing adult domestic violence.[2] It is tragic that oftentimes those who have the strongest bonds to a human being—one's own family—can perpetrate such acts of violence. The home, which should be a little heaven on earth, a shelter and safe haven filled with warmth and love, can become a place of harm, danger, and fear behind closed doors.

Such an unhealthy environment becomes a source of chronic stress, possibly resulting in disease and even death. Adults who have experienced child abuse have up to a 60 percent higher risk for diabetes.[3] Studies of childhood neglect have also found an increased risk of diabetes.[4] The current pandemic of diabetes makes such facts both startling and worrying. Who would have thought that diabetes could have anything to do with the type of relationships we have at home? But such negative physical health effects go beyond that of diabetes or the immune system. Traumatic experiences in childhood appear to have a role in cancer, cardiovascular disease, obesity and being overweight, and early death.[5] The evidence strongly suggests that if excessive stress weakens the immune system in childhood and abuse damages the delicate mechanisms of the mind, multiple physical, mental, and emotional problems may surface later in life.

Mental and Public Health Impact

Unhealthy relationships at home actually cause changes in our brain. The parts of the brain particularly affected are those that play important roles in long- and short-term memory.[6] Additionally, both children and adult victims of family violence often experience fear, shame, guilt, and stigma. Such negative emotions contribute to mental and emotional problems, including depression, bipolar disorder, and post-traumatic stress disorder in both men and women.[7]

Experiencing childhood maltreatment and poverty at an early age harms our immune system. The bodies of those who have endured such a background often show, when they become adults, an abnormal control of inflammation because of faulty immunity. They also have an increased risk for diabetes! Such immune system dysfunction appears not only in the case of child abuse, but also during adult conflict between spouses and companions, especially if it continues for some time.

Public Health Impact

Research has linked abuse and violence in all its forms not only to increased mortality but also to having a negative influence on the entire community. Globally, violence and abuse have become major problems.

The following statistics bring the health effects of violence and abuse into stark perspective: More than one in three female homicides worldwide occur at the hands of an intimate partner—often a spouse or companion.[8] Such violence commonly represents the end result of a long history of abusive relationships. Public health officials in the United States list violence among one of eight major priorities affecting the health of American citizens.

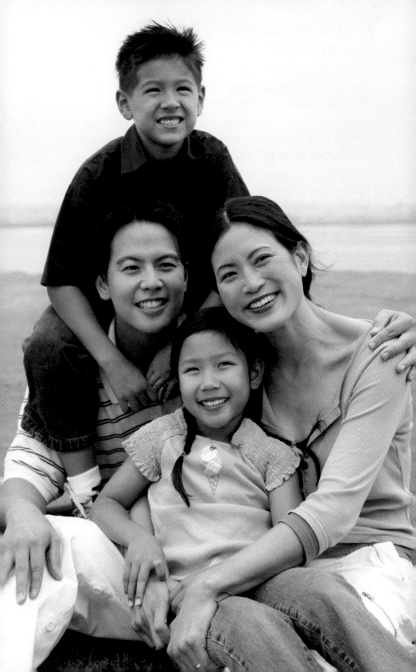

Protective Factors

Fortunately, even despite the many negative health outcomes among survivors of domestic violence, there is still hope! Not everyone who experiences abusive relationships will develop such health problems. Often described as resilience, many individuals manage to bounce back by employing effective coping mechanisms.

The good news for anyone affected by domestic violence is that such positive coping factors can help people to heal. They include cultivating wholesome emotions; learning to be flexible; developing a selfless concern for the well-being of others; having social support; and utilizing faith, religion, or spirituality.[9] In fact, studies suggest that gratitude, and forgiveness specifically,[10] can powerfully contribute to psychological resilience in the face of trauma and abuse.

Forgiveness or gratitude can be healing balms and protective factors that will enable us to deal with the disease that may result from abusive relationships. If someone has hurt you deeply and you fail to forgive them, you are allowing them to injure you a second time. An unforgiving spirit destroys our health and imprisons us in bitterness. It robs us of the joy God longs for us to have. Just as Jesus forgave those who crucified Him when they did not deserve it, so we can forgive those who have wounded us when they do not warrant it. Forgiving another does not mean that we condone their actions or justify what they did to us. Rather, forgiveness is releasing another from our condemnation when they do not deserve it, because Christ releases us from His condemnation when we do not deserve it. As the apostle Paul so clearly states, "And be kind to one another, tenderhearted, forgiving one another, even as God in Christ forgave you" (Ephesians 4:32, NKJV).

One of the questions that people have when they experience the heart wrenching trauma of abusive relationships is, "Where is God in all of this?" Pain and injustice flood the globe. At times life is just plain unfair. We live in a world of good and evil, joy and sorrow, love and hate, health and sickness. Sometimes we bring heartache upon ourselves through our own poor choices, but there are plenty of times that we have done absolutely nothing wrong, and sorrow seems to stalk us. Trauma strikes. Tears flow. Tragedy overwhelms us. But in spite of all of life's injustice, God is still near. And He will never leave us or forsake us (Hebrews 13:5). Instead, if we will let Him, He strengthens and encourages. He still heals broken hearts, sets at liberty the captives, and delivers the oppressed (Luke 4:18).

Here is an eternal biblical truth that is life transformational: God is love (1 John 4:8). His actions toward us are always and only loving ones. He would never do anything to harm us. Whatever painful, traumatic childhood experiences you may have had in the past, God did not cause them, and you are certainly not responsible for them. They were the result of harmful, destructive choices made by someone else. Do you feel guilty for something you had absolutely no control over, or blame God for it? If there is an aching void in your heart because of childhood hurts, emotional betrayal, or physical or mental abuse, Jesus understands. He was Himself betrayed and beaten, ridiculed and rejected. People lied about and laughed at Him. His enemies cursed and crucified Him. But in spite of such horrible injustices, He never lost faith in His Father's love and care. Able to understand what you have gone through, He is near to heal your heart and give you new hope for living.

Have you ever wondered about the purpose of all human relationships? Why does God give us fathers, mothers, brothers, sisters, husbands, wives, sons, daughters, and friends? Each human relationship is part of God's plan to reveal a different aspect of His love. Throughout Scripture we find Him pictured as having the qualities of a strong caring Father, a tender pitiful mother, a loving husband, an affectionate wife, a protective big brother, a listening sister, and a faithful friend. God reveals His love through the prism of human relationships.

But what if one of those relationships gets fractured through no fault of our own? What if rather than revealing God's character qualities it reflects the brokenness of sin and the destructive nature of selfishness? When we learn to trust Him, God will bypass the relationship and fill our hearts with the love we should have received from the father, mother, sister, brother, husband, wife, or friend. Read the Bible passages below and let your heart rejoice that He can supply the deepest needs of your heart:

"As a father pities his children, so the Lord pities those who fear Him" (Psalm 103:13, NKJV).

"A father of the fatherless, a defender of widows, is God in His holy habitation" (Psalm 68:5, NKJV).

"Can a woman forget her nursing child, and not have compassion on the son of her womb? Surely they may forget, yet I will not forget you" (Isaiah 49:15, NKJV).

"For your Maker is your husband, the Lord of hosts is His name; and your redeemer is the Holy One of Israel; He is called the God of the whole earth" (Isaiah 54:5, NKJV).

"But there is a friend [Jesus] who sticks closer than a brother" (Proverbs 18:24, NKJV).

These are just a sampling of Bible passages that describe the intimate relationship the Father, Son, and Holy Spirit desire to have with us. When behind closed doors our lives have been shattered, we can discover new hope in a God who will rebuild our lives and supply all that our hearts lack. Love flowing from the heart of an infinite God is healing love. In Him life is new. Through Him we can hope again, and because of Him, we can face the future with new joy.

---

1. J. K. Kiecolt-Glaser et al., "Psychosocial Enhancement of Immunocompetence in a Geriatric Population," *Health Psychology* 4 (1985): 25–41.

2. Centers for Disease Control and Prevention, "Adverse Childhood Experiences Reported by Adults," www.cdc.gov/mmwr/preview/mmwrhtml/mm5949a1.htm.

3. V. J. Felitti et al., "Relationship of Childhood Abuse and Household Dysfunction to Many of the Leading Causes of Death in Adults," *American Journal of Preventive Medicine* 14 (1998): 245–258.

4. R. D. Goodwin and M. B. Stein, "Association Between Childhood Trauma and Physical Disorders Among Adults in the United States," *Psychological Medicine* 34 (2004): 509–520.

5. Centers for Disease Control and Prevention, "Adverse Childhood Experiences Reported by Adults."

6. A. Danese and B. S. McEwen, "Adverse Childhood Experiences, Allostasis, Allostatic Load, and Age-Related Disease," *Physiology & Behavior* 106 (2012): 29–39.

7. J. McCauley et al., "Clinical Characteristics of Women With a History of Childhood Abuse: Unhealed Wounds," *Journal of the American Medical Association* 277 (1997): 1362–1368.

8. H. Stöckl et al., "The Global Prevalence of Intimate Partner Homicide: A Systematic Review," *The Lancet* 382 (2013): 859–865.

9. K. Tusaie and J. Dyer, "Resilience: A Historical Review of the Construct," *Holistic Nursing Practice* 18 (2004): 3–8.

10. A. J. Miller et al., "Gender and Forgiveness: A Meta-Analytic Review and Research Agenda," *Journal of Social and Clinical Psychology* 27 (2008): 843–876.

CHAPTER 7

YOU ARE WHAT YOU THINK

A positive attitude is life-giving: nurture it.

Have you ever questioned why at times negative thoughts flood your mind? Have you ever wondered how to turn such negative thoughts into positive ones? Have you ever noticed the impact of how you think on what you do when faced with an important moral choice or ethical dilemma?

When a group of volunteers endured two sleepless nights, army researchers found that the lack of sleep hindered the participants' ability to make decisions in the face of emotionally charged moral dilemmas.[1] Perhaps even more significant, however, was that while some volunteers changed their views of what was morally acceptable as a result of sleep deprivation, it was not universally the case. Those who, at the beginning of the study, scored high on a measure known as "emotional intelligence" did not waver on what they found morally appropriate.

This study and many others help to confirm the eternal truth in Proverbs 23:7 that as a person "thinks in his heart, so is he" (NKJV). The way we reason shapes our responses to life. Our thoughts govern what we do. Our behavior often follows what is in our minds. We act out the images that we project on the screen of our conscience. It's clear that all of us must expect to face emotionally charged moral dilemmas at least sometime in our lives. And when we do, how will we respond? At such occasions emotional intelligence may be a plus.

What Is Emotional Intelligence?

Traditionally, we have understood intelligence as the cognitive or mental capacity of a person, and the means employed to measure it is the IQ (intelligence quotient) test. Yet in 1983, developmental psychologist Howard Gardner proposed in *Frames of Mind* the theory of multiple intelligences. Instead of defining intelligence as a single logical ability, we should see it as a set of eight (later he included one more) clusters of skills: naturalist intelligence ("nature smart"), musical intelligence ("musical smart"), logical-mathematical intelligence ("number/reasoning smart"), interpersonal intelligence ("people smart"), bodily-kinesthetic intelligence ("body smart"), linguistic intelligence ("word smart"), intrapersonal intelligence ("self smart"), spatial intelligence ("picture smart"), and existential intelligence ("morality smart").[2]

Then in 1995 psychologist and science journalist Daniel Goleman launched an internationally best-selling book titled *Emotional Intelligence,* which popularized this kind of intelligence, normally defined as the sentimental capacity of the mind, or the ability to identify, assess, and control emotions. According to Goleman, emotional intelligence has five distinct aspects:[3]

1. knowing our emotions
2. managing our emotions
3. recognizing emotions in others
4. managing relationships with others
5. motivating ourselves to achieve our goals

All of them are important, for we always need to decipher and manage emotions.

The Role of Emotional Intelligence

Emotional intelligence (EQ or EI) is not related merely to decision-making. Studies show that while the job a person gets after graduating from college might reflect their IQ, how far they advance in that job bears little relationship to it.[4] It's not even connected to their grades in school. Rather, it's related to their EQ. Our success and happiness in life are more closely associated with EQ than with any other form of intelligence.

A variety of scientific studies has shown that increasing a person's EQ will prevent or treat depression, phobias, obsessive-compulsive disorder, post-traumatic stress disorder, anorexia, bulimia, and addictions such as alcoholism.[5] The 12-step program of Alcoholics Anonymous, for example, has achieved remarkable success, but it is four times more successful if combined with a program to enhance emotional intelligence.

What about persons who don't necessarily have an addiction or a specific disease?

Enhancing EQ will help those individuals to think more clearly and communicate more effectively. It fosters unity in group settings, reduces polarizing statements, and promotes a happier life.

Influences on Emotional Intelligence

Researchers have done extensive studies during the past decade on what can influence EQ. Our genetic makeup, childhood experiences, and current level of emotional support all play a role. So does what we eat.

Bonnie Beezhold has shown that a plant-based diet is associated with healthier mood states in both men and women.[6] Switching to a vegetarian diet will reduce levels of stress, anxiety, and depression, apparently because plant foods don't have arachidonic acid, an inflammatory fat present largely in meat and fish.

Our activities have an impact on both our IQ and EQ The more entertainment television watched, the lower the creativity and one's grades.[7] In addition, a lack of emotional control—including an increase in violent and sexual crimes—results.[8] Entertainment Internet, videos, and video games also have an adverse effect. As the apostle Paul stated: "By beholding we become changed" (see 2 Corinthians 3:18).

The most important influence on EQ, however, is what we believe. Our beliefs—that is, our evaluations of events, the way we think about problems, our silent (or sometimes not-so-silent) self-talk—largely

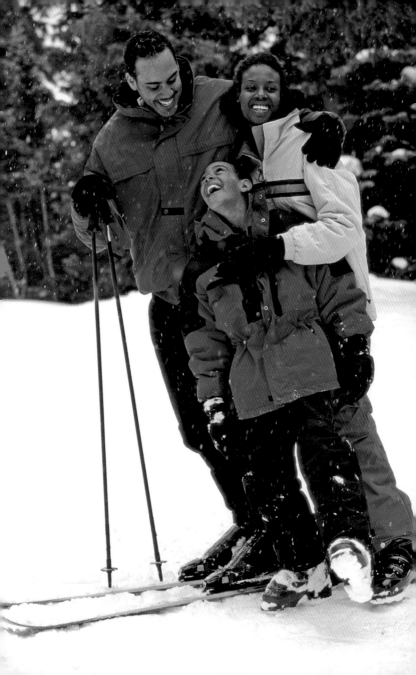

shape our emotions. Thus our beliefs have much more to do with how we feel than what is actually happening in our lives.

Set Free

If the thoughts are wrong, the feelings will be wrong—and thoughts and feelings combined make up the personal character. But the good news is that reconstructing our thinking *will* change us. The Bible says, "Be transformed by the renewing of your mind" (Romans 12:2, NIV). We not only have to recognize distorted thoughts, but we must correct them and replace them with true and accurate ones that find their source in God.

How then can we safeguard and improve our emotional intelligence? By eating healthy foods; getting adequate sleep; avoiding bad entertainment on the Internet, television, and in movies; and rejecting cognitive distortions: self-magnification, emotion-based reasoning, overgeneralization, and so forth.[9] We must fill our minds with accurate and true thoughts, ones derived from an understanding of God's plan for our lives. Then, Christ says, "you shall know the truth, and the truth shall make you free" (John 8:32, NKJV).

The way to get rid of negative thoughts is by replacing them with positive ones. Self-defeating, depressing thoughts will rush into our minds. But at those times, the counsel of the apostle Paul is extremely helpful: "Set your mind on things above, not on things on earth. For you died, and your life is hidden with Christ in God. When Christ who is our life appears, you will also appear with Him in glory" (Colossians 3:2–4, NKJV). Notice this divine instruction carefully. First it counsels us to "set our minds on things above." We might rephrase it this way: "Choose to fill your mind with the reality of divine truth. Do not allow the distortions the devil brings to you to shape your thinking."

"Setting our minds on things above" makes a major difference in our thought processes for two significant reasons. First, we sense anew that "our lives are hidden with Christ in God." In Him we are affirmed and accepted. And in Him we are safe and secure. He is our refuge and strength. On the cross Jesus triumphed over all of the forces of evil. His victory is ours (Colossians 2:15). Nothing can rip us out of His hands (John 10:27, 28). Nothing can separate us from His love (Romans 8:35–39). And nothing can rob us of our deep inner peace and joy, if by faith we daily grasp the reality that our real life is in the protection of Jesus and God.

Second, "setting our minds on things above" is powerfully life-transformational because "when Christ who is our life appears" at the Second Coming, we will join Him in glory. This is hope and encouragement beyond anything that might trouble and harass us. Jesus is coming again to take us home. One day sorrow, suffering, disease, and depression will be over. Oppression and injustice will fade into the eternal past. In Christ, through Christ, and because of Christ, we can think positive, hopeful, joyous thoughts today and throughout all eternity.

1. W.D.S. Killgore et al., "The Effects of 53 Hours of Sleep Deprivation on Moral Judgment," *Sleep* 30 (2007): 345–352.

2. See Howard Gardner, *Frames of Mind: The Theory of Multiple Intelligences* (New York: Basic Books, 2003).

3. See Daniel Goleman, *Emotional Intelligence: Why It Can Matter More Than IQ* (New York: Bantam Books, 1995).

4. M. D. Aydin et al., "The Impact of IQ and EQ on Pre-eminent Achievement in Organizations: Implications for the Hiring Decisions of HRM Specialists," *International Journal of Human Resource Management* 16 (2005): 701–719.

5. L. M. Ito et al., "Cognitive-Behavioral Therapy in Social Phobia," *Revista Brasileira de Psiquiatria* 30 (2008): S96–101; T. D. Borkovec and E. Costello, "Efficacy of Applied Relaxation and Cognitive-Behavioral Therapy in the Treatment of Generalized Anxiety Disorder," *Journal of Consulting and Clinical Psychology* 61 (1993): 611–619; G. A. Fava et al., "Six-Year Outcome of Cognitive Behavior Therapy for Prevention of Recurrent Depression," *American Journal of Psychiatry* 161 (2004): 1872–1876.

6. B. L. Beezhold, C. S. Johnston, and D. R. Daigle, "Vegetarian Diets Are Associated With Healthy Mood States: A Cross-Sectional Study in Seventh Day Adventist Adults," *Nutrition Journal* 9 (2010), www.nutritionj.com/content/pdf/1475-2891-9-26.pdf.

7. I. Sharif and J. D. Sargent, "Association Between Television, Movie, and Video Game Exposure and School Performance," *Pediatrics* 118 (2006): e1061–1070.

8. L. R. Huesmann et al., "Longitudinal Relations Between Children's Exposure to TV Violence and Their Aggressive and Violent Behavior in Young Adulthood: 1977-1992," *Developmental Psychology* 39 (2003): 201–221; B. J. Bushman and C. A. Anderson, "Media Violence and the American Public: Scientific Facts Versus Media Misinformation," *American Psychologist* 56 (2001): 477–489.

9. Neil Nedley, *The Lost Art of Thinking: How to Improve Emotional Intelligence and Achieve Peak Mental Performance* (Ardmore, Okla.: Nedley Pub., 2011).

CHAPTER 8

HOPE BEYOND DEPRESSION

There is a better day coming: anticipate it.

Depression is a global problem that can affect anyone anywhere. Statistics reveal that more than 350 million people of all ages suffer from it. The leading cause of disability worldwide, it is a major part of the global burden of disease. Those who study the patterns of disease predict that such figures will only increase in the future.

The World Health Organization describes depression as "a common mental disorder," characterized by sadness, loss of interest or pleasure, feelings of guilt or low self-worth, disturbed sleep or appetite, feelings of tiredness, and poor concentration.[1] "At its worst, depression can lead to suicide." An estimated 1 million people die from depression-related deaths each year. This is even more disturbing when we realize that a number of positive principles and effective treatments can make a major difference for people dealing with depression.

Even a better standard of living does not ensure happiness. "Based on detailed interviews with over 89,000 people, [study] results showed that 15 percent of the population from high-income countries, compared to 11 percent for low or middle-income countries, were likely to get depression over their lifetime, with 5.5 percent having had depression in the last year."[2] As we see, money is not a solution to disappointment, discouragement, and despair.

The same research shows that women are "twice as likely to suffer depression as men, and the loss of a partner, whether from death, divorce or separation, was a main contributing factor."[3] The cause of depression is not the same for everyone. For some, it is a genetic problem that affects the balance of chemicals (neurotransmitters) in the brain. For others, a stressful life event, such as the death of a loved one, losing a job, a divorce, or some equally distressing life event, may trigger it. In many cases depression occurs as a result of the combination of both the chemical imbalance and a triggering event. Whatever the cause, whether it is a chemical upset in the brain or the heartache of some major life event, depression can harm a person's life and needs effective solutions.

A Serious Condition

Depression can be very disabling. Millions of people live in the dark shadow of sadness, gloom, and hopelessness, and often struggle with feelings of inadequacy and worthlessness. While there are degrees of depression—and we all experience minor versions of it—almost 22 women out of every 100 will have an episode or more of major depression during their lifetime. That is almost double the chance of such an event occurring in men. Approximately 13 out of every 100 men during their lifetime cope with some form of depression. Children under the age of ten may also experience depression, though the gender difference is not apparent until the reproductive years during and after adolescence. Once they pass menopause, though, women become less prone to depression.

Multiple factors make women more susceptible to stress-induced depression than men. They also are about four times more prone to seasonal-affective depression than men. It is the form of depression that occurs in areas where winter daylight hours are very short. People wake up and go to work in the dark and return home in darkness, and have little exposure to sunlight. Yet another factor that may influence the onset of depression is the hormonal fluctuations of the reproductive years. They may well affect neurotransmitters in the brain, increasing vulnerability to depression.

Women in many cultures do not enjoy equal status with men, something that could also play a role in depression. The demands placed

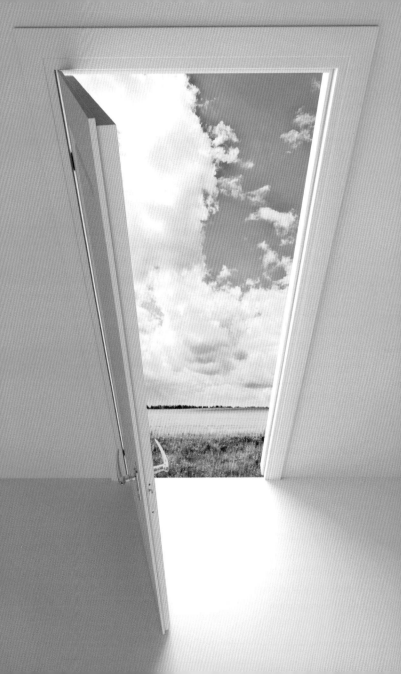

upon women to produce children or to regulate family size mean that they often carry disproportionate responsibilities and accountability for reproductive function. Infertility or a miscarriage may be viewed as a failure to fulfill their role. Oral contraceptives can carry a potential for depression in susceptible women. Hormonal factors may play a cyclical (occurring monthly) role or during the postpartum state following childbirth. Whatever the causes, women with depression need and deserve serious and compassionate care.

The symptoms of depression vary from person to person. Persistent tiredness and loss of energy are common complaints among those suffering from it. Depressed individuals may suffer from loss of concentration and become indecisive. Feelings of guilt and low self-worth often persist for weeks and even months at a time. Some may experience difficulty sleeping or, on the other hand, sleep more than normal. Many find themselves waking up early. Persons suffering from depression tend to lose interest in daily activities. They may struggle with recurring thoughts of death and suicide. Changes in eating patterns may cause either weight loss or weight gain (a change of more than 5 percent of body weight in a month). In severe cases, individuals with depression lose interest in eating and no longer find pleasure in any of life's activities, including social relationships.

Society needs to recognize that the major depressive disorders are as much a disease as the more physical ones, such as diabetes or hepatitis. Ill-advised comments such as "pull yourself together" or "get a grip" reflect either a lack of knowledge or, even more sadly, the ignorance of the one making them. Such statements may cause further pain, heartache, and a worsening of the depression.

Treatment of Depression

A person with a major depressive illness will need professional help. It is dangerous and ill-advised for even well-meaning but untrained health enthusiasts to try to interfere in the life of a person struggling with the condition.

There exist a number of approaches to the treatment of major depression. Anyone who has symptoms of depression must seek the aid of an informed and qualified health professional. Careful evaluation will help to determine the precise form of treatment needed. Severe cases may call for hospital admission. Along with medication, such programs will provide counseling and a helpful approach such as cognitive behavioral therapy. Patients may often take medication for a number of months and, sometimes, require repeated treatments.

Minor depression in men and women will often respond to programs of exercise. The Harvard Medical School reports some encouraging news about dealing with depression: A review of studies stretching back to 1981 concluded that "regular exercise can improve mood in people with mild to moderate depression—and may even play a supporting role in treating severe depression."

The report further states that the "study published in *Archives of Internal Medicine* assigned 156 depressed patients to an aerobic exercise program, the SSRI sertraline (Zoloft [a kind of antidepressant]), or both. At the 16-week mark 60 to 70 percent of the people in all three groups no longer had major depression. In fact, group scores on two rating scales of depression were essentially the same." "A study published in 2005 . . . found that walking fast for about 35 minutes a day five times a week or 60 minutes a day three times a week significantly improved symptoms in people with mild to moderate depression."[4]

If you are feeling a little down, get out, take a walk, and breathe deeply. While you do so, meditate on God's goodness and ask Him to fill your mind with positive thoughts.

Another factor in dealing with depression involves the food we eat. The Mayo Clinic reports that diet may contribute to depression: "Some preliminary research suggests that having a poor diet can make you more vulnerable to depression. Researchers in Britain looked at depression and diet in more than 3,000 middle-aged office workers over the course of five years. They found that people who ate a junk food diet—one that was high in processed meat, chocolates, sweet desserts, fried food, refined cereals, and high-fat dairy products—were more likely to report symptoms of depression."⁵

In other words, when you eat your veggies, you are benefitting your brain as well as your body. Now, don't misunderstand us—we are not suggesting that consuming a carrot a day will keep you singing all the time. Depression is a complex subject, but a healthy diet is part of an overall wellness program that will assist in reducing the problem.

Some general health habits can also be effective:

- Eat healthfully of a well-balanced plant-based diet.
- Have regular sleep and rest routines.
- Exercise regularly outdoors.
- Cultivate meaningful relationships with family and friends.
- Trust in the power and grace of our loving heavenly Father.
- Change your pattern of thought, trying to focus your mind on possibilities and positive things.
- Seek professional help if you experience symptoms of depression for prolonged periods, and then follow the prescribed treatment of qualified health personnel.

One of the strongest antidotes for depression is social support. Warm, loving relationships, close friendships, and strong family ties make all the difference. If you are feeling down, confide in a friend, share your burden with someone you can trust. You do not need to bear it alone. In fact, Jesus Himself invites us to bring our heaviest burdens to Him. He says, "Come to Me, all you who labor and are heavy laden, and I will give you rest" (Matthew 11:28, NKJV). When dealing with depression, proper stress management can be helpful, as well as a balanced spiritual relationship with God.

A High Note

So let's end the chapter on a high note. Cynthia (pseudonym), a professional colleague of one of the authors of this book, experienced prolonged and deep depression. But in time, as she followed some of the counsels given here, she broke free from the despair that enslaved her. Here is her counsel to anyone experiencing a similar situation: "If you are depressed for a prolonged period of time, get help. Don't rule out medication. Medication can break down the wall of darkness that surrounds you, and this breakthrough will give you the strength you need to make lifestyle changes that could assist your recovery. Find a good, highly recommended doctor. Share your struggle with someone else, and ask that person to pray for you.

"If your depression is a life struggle, feed on the Word of God," she advises. "Read and memorize 'joy' texts, such as Nehemiah 8:10, Psalms 34, 40, and 66, and the book of Philippians. Begin a 'joy journal' in which you give God thanks for five things each night before you go to sleep. Feed your mind with good things. Highlight texts in your Bible that talk of joy, rejoicing, gladness, and praise, so that you can claim those texts each day." Finally, she always likes to quote a phrase written by a Hebrew poet: "Because You have been my help, therefore in the shadow of Your wings I will rejoice" (Psalm 63:7, NKJV).

Remember this eternal truth: it is a law of the mind that it gradually adapts itself to the subjects you allow it to dwell on. Fill your mind with positive thoughts. Meditate upon God's Word. Claim His promises as your own. Believe that Jesus, the light of the world, will illuminate your darkness. Do not accept lies about yourself. A valuable child of God, you mean more to Him than you will ever know. Understanding our worth in His sight and His care for us will help us to thrive!

1. World Health Organization, "Depression," Fact Sheet No. 369, www.who.int/mediacentre/factsheets/fs369/en/index.html.
2. BioMed Central, "Global Depression Statistics," www.sciencedaily.com/releases/2011/07/110725202240.htm.
3. Ibid.
4. Harvard Health Publications, *Understanding Depression* (Boston: Harvard Medical School, 2008), www.hrccatalog.hrrh.on.ca/InmagicGenie/DocumentFolder/understanding%20depression.pdf.
5. Mayo Clinic, "Diseases and Conditions: Can a Junk Food Diet Increase Your Risk of Depression?" www.mayoclinic.org/diseases-conditions/depression/expert-answers/depression-and-diet/faq-20058241.

CHAPTER 9

BREAKING FREE

Balance is the pathway to success: seek it.

According to the "Global Status Report on Alcohol and Health" released by the World Health Organization in Geneva in February 2011:[1]

- Approximately 2.5 million people die from alcohol-related causes each year.
- Fifty-five percent of adults have consumed it.
- Almost 4 percent of all deaths worldwide are related to alcohol through injuries, cancer, cardiovascular diseases, and liver cirrhosis.
- Globally, 6.2 percent of male deaths involve alcohol.

The World Health Organization report also revealed that worldwide in 2005, 6.13 liters of pure alcohol were consumed per person age 15 years or older. The amount appeared to be stable in the Americas and the European, Eastern Mediterranean, and Western Pacific regions. However, the researchers noted marked rises in Africa and Southeast Asia. Health risk increases even more with binge drinking or when people drink solely to get drunk. Definitions of binge drinking vary, but in the United States health officials consider more than five consecutive drinks for a male and more than four for a female to be binge drinking. The practice of binge drinking is exploding in many parts of the world.

Alcohol consumption leads to tens of thousands of preventable deaths each year. "In the European Union [EU], alcohol accounts for about 120,000 premature deaths per year: 1 in 7 in men and 1 in 13 in women," says another report of the World Health Organization.[2] Such worrying facts place alcohol alongside tobacco as one of the world's leading preventable causes of death and disability.[3] No ordinary commodity, alcohol is very dangerous.

Alcohol Addiction

Of every 100 people who drink alcohol, 13 will develop alcoholism during their lifetimes. If there's a first-degree relative (e.g., father, mother, uncle, aunt, grandparent) who has suffered from alcohol dependence, the likelihood doubles. But should experimentation with alcohol begin under the age of 14 years, the chance of becoming addicted increases to 40 percent-plus![4]

We need to educate children about the dangers of alcohol from an early age. Parents and others must foster healthy relationships and connectedness from an early age. Such social support develops resilience and promotes healthful choices. An additional layer of protection for both young and old is a vital, personal faith in God.

Why is faith so important when dealing with addictions? For two very significant reasons. First, an understanding that our bodies are not fun houses, but the temple of the living God makes all the difference. The Christ who both created us and redeemed us longs to live in us through His Holy Spirit. The apostle Paul's words echo down the corridors of time: "Or do you not know that your body is the temple of the Holy Spirit who is in you, whom you have from God, and you are not your own? For you were bought at a price; therefore glorify God in your body and in your spirit which are God's" (1 Corinthians 6:19, 20, NKJV).

The second reason faith makes so much difference in our ability to overcome destructive habits is that when we choose to surrender our weak, wavering wills to God, He strengthens us to be able to overcome destructive lifestyle habits. The apostle John states it succinctly:

"For whatever is born of God overcomes the world. And this is the victory that has overcome the world—our faith" (1 John 5:4, NKJV). Our loving heavenly Father desires that each one of us live a life free from crippling addictions that predispose us to life-threatening diseases such as heart disease and cancer.

Alcohol and Cancer

Cancer is one of the leading causes of death worldwide. Researchers in the European Union, where cancer has become the second-most-common cause of death (with about 2.5 million cancer deaths per year), estimate that alcohol consumption directly causes 10 percent of cancers in men and 3 percent of those in women. Avoiding alcohol could prevent approximately 30 percent of total cancers in the European Union.[5] Worldwide, we find strong evidence that alcohol triggers breast cancer in women and colon cancer in both men and women. There appears no safe limit/dose of alcohol that will avoid its carcinogenic (cancer-causing) effect. It is, therefore, clearly dangerous for anyone to recommend alcohol use to enhance health, as some are doing for possible cardiac benefits.

Alcohol and Society

It's well known that alcohol use lies behind accidents of all kinds, such as road fatalities, as well as domestic violence, murder, rape, and other criminal activities. Alcohol is also the leading cause of preventable mental retardation in the world. It easily crosses the placenta and damages the developing brain of the unborn baby. As a result, there is no safe level of alcohol consumption during pregnancy.

Alcohol and Heart Health

For the past 30 years, some have promoted alcohol as "heart healthy" and protective against coronary artery disease. Much has appeared in popular and scientific publications on the subject. But the many contradictory results of the various studies may be for a wide variety of reasons. Prominent researchers have suggested that some or all of the apparent cardiac protective effect of moderate drinking may be the result of other factors.[6] Differences in health status, education, and socioeconomic status of the individuals studied have added even more confusion in interpreting the data. For example, a number of the subjects included in the nondrinking group had been drinkers prior to the studies being done and had stopped using alcohol for health reasons.[7] A growing number of researchers attribute the better heart health outcomes among the moderate drinkers not to alcohol, but to their average health status and healthful lifestyle in other behaviors, such as exercise and diet that were superior to those of the nondrinkers studied.[8]

Taking into account all the definite health risks related to alcohol, it doesn't make sense to promote its use for heart health, especially when other proven and safe ways to prevent heart disease exist, such as daily exercise and a healthful diet.

Killer Tobacco

Another killer is tobacco. Every day more than 1 billion people smoke or chew tobacco, and 15,000 die daily from tobacco-related diseases.[9] Most of those deaths could be avoided if people did not smoke, as well as still more if we eradicated secondhand smoke. The bottom line is: If you smoke, you put yourself at risk.

Tobacco is a lethal and freely available poison marketed in various forms. It's smoked, chewed, inhaled, used electronically, and even dissolved in water (*shisha*). All forms are harmful, substantially increasing the risk of disease and even death. Tobacco kills up to half its users!

- Tobacco contributes to the deaths of nearly 6 million people each year. Six hundred thousand of them are nonsmokers exposed to secondhand smoke.
- Nearly 80 percent of the world's 1 billion smokers live in low- and middle-income countries.
- Consumption of tobacco products continues to increase globally.

- Approximately one person dies every six seconds as a result of tobacco-related causes.
- Up to half of current users will eventually die of a tobacco-related disease.

Tobacco is a gradual killer with a lag of several years between starting to use tobacco and when the user's health deteriorates. It's one of the most significant public health threats the world has ever faced, not only killing the user but often negatively affecting the health of, or even killing, those exposed to secondhand tobacco smoke. Tobacco smoke contains more than 2,000 chemicals and substances. At least 250 of them are known to be harmful, and more than 50 cause cancer.

Secondhand smoke by definition is the smoke that fills restaurants, offices, homes, and any enclosed space in which tobacco products burn, including cigarettes, cigars, pipes, *bidis,* and water pipes (*shisha*). With no safe level of exposure, it's a proven cause of cardiovascular and respiratory disease in adults, including lung cancer and coronary heart disease. In babies it can cause sudden infant death syndrome. Children in contact with secondhand smoke have more upper- and lower-respiratory infections.

Furthermore, tobacco is a "gateway drug."[10] Those who use it place themselves at risk of using and becoming addicted to other drugs, such as marijuana, methamphetamine, cocaine, and heroin.

Both alcohol and tobacco are extremely dangerous. Scientific evidence and public health statistics show them to be leading killers in the world today. It's a personal choice whether to use tobacco, alcohol, or other harmful, health-destroying substances, but our choices have consequences.

The facts certainly speak for themselves. We were created for something better than to experience preventable diseases as a result of our poor decisions. Remember that it is never too late to begin making positive lifestyle choices, and when we do, God comes immediately to our aid to empower our decisions. What we could never accomplish on our own we can through His strength.

Enemy Number One

As far back as 1971 then-president Richard Nixon stated that "America's public enemy number one in the United States is drug abuse. In order to fight and defeat this enemy, it is necessary to wage a new, all-out offensive."[11] If it was true at that time, it is much more so today, and the same reality applies also to other countries.

Because of its illegal nature, we can have no precise statistics about the size of the illicit drug industry. Experts have estimated it at $300 billion, $400 billion, and even $1 trillion per year.[12] In 2010, United Nations Office on Drugs and Crime calculated that between 153 million and 300 million people ages 15 to 64 took drugs during the previous year, with a higher prevalence of cannabis (marijuana) followed by amphetamine-type stimulants. As a rule, the use of illicit drugs by males far exceeds that by females, who, more often resort to tranquillizers and sedatives.[13]

It has been estimated that only 20 percent of problem drug users receive treatment for their dependence. The tragedies resulting from such dangerous consumption are staggering. The number of deaths as a consequence of drugs has been calculated to be between 99,000 and 253,000. In some countries great numbers of murders are drug-related. For example, the Mexican government estimates that 90 percent of the killings in the country have connections with drugs. While that may be an extreme case, it still tells us much about the malignant potential of illicit drugs.[14]

The impact of drug use on one's health is beyond description. Many think about it only when a celebrity such as Philip Seymour Hoffman dies. According to the medical examiner, the Oscar-winning actor was killed "by a toxic mix of drugs." However, numerous ordinary people get sick and die every day as a result of drug abuse.

Drugs affect almost every organ of the body. They can weaken the immune system, increasing susceptibility to infections; cause cardiovascular problems, including abnormal heart rate, heart attacks, and infections of the blood vessels and heart valves; provoke nausea, vomiting, and abdominal pain; damage the liver; trigger stroke; alter brain chemistry, leading to substance dependency; do permanent brain damage; affect memory, attention, and decision-making; induce paranoia, aggressiveness, hallucinations, depression, and addiction; and "may pose various risks for pregnant women and their babies."[15]

Fortunately the drug users and their families don't need to face the challenge alone. Many treatment centers and support services can help. Narcotics Anonymous is one of them. Its vision is that "every addict in the world has the chance to experience our message in his or her own language and culture and find the opportunity for a new way of life."[16] With human and divine help, victory is possible.

True Balance in Living

You may be struggling with the shackles of addiction to alcohol, tobacco, drugs, overwork, pornography, media addiction, or just living an unbalanced life. Few feelings can match the sheer desperation of attempting to give up something and failing, and then continuing to try and still failing. Habits form easily, but are difficult to break. In fact, sheer grit and willpower ("won't power," if you will!) are not enough to gain victory over enslaving habits and addictions. We need help.

For additional information on recovery ideas, visit these Web sites: www.AdventistRecovery.org and http://FactsWithHope.org.

---

1. Available online at www.who.int/substance_abuse/publications/global_alcohol_report/en.
2. "Status Report on Alcohol and Health in 35 European Countries 2013," www.euro.who.int /en/publications/abstracts/status-report-on-alcohol-and-health-in-35-european-countries-2013.
3. Thomas Babor et al., *Alcohol: No Ordinary Commodity,* 2nd ed. (New York: Oxford University Press, 2010), 70.
4. Richard K. Ries et al., *Principles of Addiction Medicine,* 4th ed. (Philadelphia: Lippincott Williams and Wilkins, 2009).
5. EuroCare, European Alcohol Policy Alliance, "Alcohol and Cancer—the Forgotten Link," www.eurocare.org/library/latest_news/alcohol_and_cancer_the_forgotten_link.
6. Timothy S. Naimi et al., "Cardiovascular Risk Factors and Confounders Among Nondrinking and Moderate-Drinking U.S. Adults," *American Journal of Preventive Medicine* 28 (2005): 369–373.
7. Kaye Middleton Fillmore et al., "Moderate Alcohol Use and Reduced Mortality Risk: Systematic Error in Prospective Studies," *Addiction Research and Theory* 14 (2006): 101–132.
8. B. Hansel et al., "Relationship Between Alcohol Intake, Health and Social Status, and Cardiovascular Risk Factors in the Urban Paris-Ile-de-France Cohort," *European Journal of Clinical Nutrition* 64 (2010): 561–568.
9. Robert Beaglehole et al., "Priority Actions for the Noncommunicable Disease Crisis," *Lancet* 377 (2011): 1438–1447.
10. World Health Organization, "Tobacco," Fact Sheet No. 339; www.who.int/mediacentre

/factsheets/fs339/en/index.html. See also Omar Sharey et al., *The Tobacco Atlas,* 3rd ed. (Atlanta: American Cancer Society, 2009).

11. Richard Nixon, "Remarks About an Intensified Program for Drug Abuse Prevention and Control," June 17, 1971. Available online by John T. Woolley and Gerhard Peters, the American Presidency Project, at www.presidency.ucsb.edu/ws/?pid=3047. For a chronology of America's drug war, see www.pbs.org/wgbh/pages/frontline/shows/drugs/cron/.

12. See www.unodc.org/pdf/WDR_2005/volume_1_chap2.pdf.

13. Data available at www.unodc.org/documents/data-and-analysis/WDR2012/WDR_2012_Chapter1.pdf.

14. Ibid.

15. Gateway Foundation, "Effects of Drug Abuse and Addiction," http://recovergateway.org/resources/individuals/drug-addiction-effects/.

16. Visit the Web site www.na.org/.

CHAPTER 10

REST FOR OUR RESTLESSNESS

Rest is the remedy for fatigue: cherish it.

Tales come from eighteenth- and nineteenth-century England about how factory managers stole time from their workers. The managers would simply push the hands of the clocks back as the day progressed, forcing the unfortunate employees to work longer hours without extra pay. Another ploy involved having the minute hand move in three-minute intervals during the lunch hour instead of one, thus shortening the break. Such practices robbed the workers of the one commodity that we can never make up, and that is time.

We may lose money in the stock market or in other bad investments, but we can sometimes get it back. Or if we lose our health, we may some-times regain it through proper medical attention, diet, and exercise. But time lost or stolen—whether one minute, one day, one week, whatever—is gone forever. In the movie *In Time* (2011) society controls the aging process in order to avoid overpopulation. Having much money, rich indi-viduals can purchase a longer life span than those who are poor. However, what is possible in fiction is impossible in real life. Nobody can buy time.

The clock ticks onward regardless of what we do. From every direc-tion forces work to take our time from us just as surely as a pickpocket will our wallets. Faster phones, faster electronic tablets, faster Internet connections, and faster computers have not, it seems, resulted in more time for us. On the contrary, it's one of the sad facts of the modern world that the faster we do things the less time we have for ourselves. And although lack of time is a great ailment of modern life, a powerful antidote to our modern dilemma actually comes from antiquity. It's called Sabbath, and it is, along with proper sleep, one of the best ways to find rest for human restlessness.

Refuge

In parts of the world in which hurricanes, tornadoes, and tsunamis occur, people build shelters. Such shelters exist for one reason: to give people refuge from storms, particularly tornadoes. But there's a problem: we have to get to the shelter. If we are not near one and the storm strikes, we can be without refuge. No such shelter ever seeks us out—we have to go to it.

God, however, has created one that, instead of us having to rush to it, it comes to us! At 1,000 miles an hour (the speed of the earth's rotation), the Sabbath circles the globe. Arriving on one sundown, leaving on the next, the seventh-day Sabbath washes over the planet, bringing with it to our homes and lives a refuge from the world's ceaseless demands upon us and upon our time. This refuge, this rest, is so important that God offers it to us once a week, without exception. Our Sabbath rest is a symbol of our trust in our loving Creator, who cares for us more than we can imagine. On Sabbath we find shelter and protection from life's cares, anxieties, and problems.

The Sabbath symbolizes our rest in the One who loves us more than we can imagine. Abraham Heschel, a prominent Jewish author, described the Sabbath as a "palace in time."[1] Once a week God's heavenly palace descends from heaven to earth for 24 hours and our Creator opens to us the glory of His presence. Free from earth's perplexities and the worrisome burdens of daily living, we are shut in with Him in our Sabbath sanctuary of refuge. God not only invites us into His Sabbath rest, but commands us to worship and to cease from our work. He knows that a life of incessant hurry and constant work will break down our life forces, weaken our immune systems, and so absorb our focus that we would forget about Him. Along with the commandments against killing, stealing, and adultery, we find the commandment to rest. That tells us how important it is for our general well-being. But the rest that our Lord is speaking about is much more than a physical one, although it surely includes sleep. It is the total rest of mind, body, and spirit in the context of His love and care for us.

Sleep and the Sabbath Rest

Without question, among all the things the Sabbath is about and all the things it brings to us, rest is central. Even the name itself in Hebrew, *Shabbat,* comes from a verb that means "to cease, to rest." Yet no matter how crucial the Sabbath rest can be, in and of itself it's just not enough. Resting one day a week, however beneficial spiritually, mentally, and physically it is to us, would be insufficient without another kind of rest—that of sleep.

God doesn't come right out and command us to get enough sleep, as He does for us with our Sabbath rest. He doesn't need to because our bodies themselves, if we will listen to them, give us the commands. It's up to us whether we'll heed them or not. In a sense, as the Sabbath always comes to us, sleep does the same.

Of course, just as violating God's commands brings negative consequences, ignoring what our body tells us will as well. In 2011, a Chinese man died after a three-day marathon he spent in front of the computer in a cybercafé almost without eating and drinking. Two years later, in December 2013, Mira Diran, a young employee of the advertising agency Young & Rubicam in Indonesia, worked continuously for three days. She used energy drinks to keep awake. But the price she paid for her extravagant dedication was death.

It's amazing how bleak and gloomy the world can seem when seen through eyes drooping from sleep-deprived exhaustion. On the other hand, the sense of rebirth and renewal after a long night of deep sleep is totally refreshing. After all, if God created human beings to work (Genesis 2:15), He also created them to rest. And between the rest of the Sabbath and that of sleep, and the blessing of balanced, productive work; we can enjoy optimal physical, spiritual, and mental well-being. Sabbath and sleep are the true rest for human restlessness.

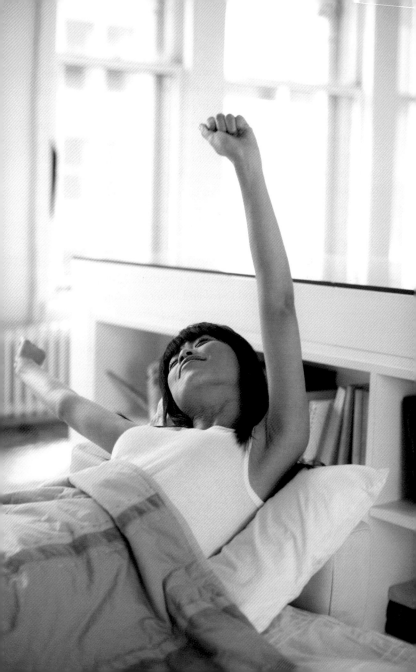

Sleep

Scientific research is clear: as human beings we need sleep. Without enough of it, we cannot function properly. Everyone, whether they will admit it or not, knows how important sleep is. Yet despite years of study, it still remains a mystery. Exactly what it is, what it does, and why it affects our bodies and minds the way it does are questions that still need many answers. We do know that sleep is essential to health and well-being. While it does not guarantee that you won't get sick, the lack of it means that sooner or later you will.

How much sleep is enough? The answer varies, because people, their health, their work habits, their age, and their metabolism vary. For practical purposes, most people need about eight hours of sleep a night (some studies put the range between seven and nine hours). It is the optimal amount necessary to experience sleep's full benefits. Besides just helping us feel rested and better emotionally and physically, sleep helps fight off infection, prevents diabetes, and reduces the risk of heart disease, obesity, and high blood pressure.

"Sleep health is a particular concern for individuals with chronic disabilities and disorders such as arthritis, kidney disease, pain, human immunodeficiency virus (HIV), epilepsy, Parkinson's disease, and depression. Among older adults, the cognitive and medical consequences of untreated sleep disorders decrease health-related quality of life, contribute to functional limitations and loss of independence, and are associated with an increased risk of death from any cause."[2]

Sleepless Around the World

Despite laborsaving devices, jet travel, and high-speed Internet, we are not getting enough sleep. You would think that with everything being done faster, we'd have more time to rest and relax. But many around the world are sleeping less than the recommended seven to nine hours. In addition, an increasing number of people have sleep problems, with many millions suffering from some type of chronic sleep disorder.

Lack of sleep leads to decreased performance during the day.

Reducing sleep by even one and a half hours, even for just one night, results in a drop of daytime alertness by as much as 32 percent. Furthermore, lack of sleep weakens memory and cognitive skills. And who hasn't experienced the added stress caused by someone's crankiness or irritability from not getting enough sleep? Workplace accidents are twice as likely to happen in cases in which one of the workers didn't get sufficient sleep. The National Highway Traffic Safety Administration (NHTSA) estimates that each year drowsy driving leads to at least 100,000 automobile crashes, 71,000 injuries, and 1,550 fatalities just within the United States. Because problems caused by lack of sleep affect those around us as well, it becomes, therefore, our responsibility to get adequate sleep and rest.

Tips for Better Sleeping

Although some people have serious sleep issues that require medical attention, here are a few simple hints that can help most of us have the restful sleep we need:

- Take your sleep seriously. Be intentional about getting adequate sleep and rest each night.
- Develop regular sleep patterns. Our bodies work on rhythms, so try to go to bed at the same time every night and get up at the same time, even on weekends.
- Regular physical exercise (the amount your doctor recommends for you) can be very beneficial in helping you get a good night's sleep. When you exercise, your body burns up energy, and sleep is the best way (along with eating proper food) to restore it. "The sleep of a labouring man is sweet" (Ecclesiastes 5:12, KJV).
- Do not go to sleep on a full stomach. Develop the routine of a light evening meal and avoid food for at least two hours prior to going to bed.
- Avoid caffeinated beverages, as caffeine is a stimulant and may keep you awake.

- Avoid stressful situations before going to sleep. Take the TV out of the bedroom permanently. Resolve family disagreements during daylight hours, not at bedtime.
- Focus on spiritual things and claim God's promises about trusting and resting in Him. "Rest in the Lord, and wait patiently for him" (Psalm 37:7, NKJV). Many people find it extremely beneficial to read from Psalms before they go to sleep each evening. The psalms tend to bring calm to our lives and a peace to our souls. They relax the mind and prepare it for sleep.

Weekly Rest

Sleep is not the only component of our overall need of rest. As we have seen, God commanded the weekly Sabbath rest, because He knew that, unless ordered to do it, we wouldn't take the necessary rest. If people, so driven by the desire to get ahead, to earn more money, to learn more, don't allow themselves even enough physical sleep, who would keep the Sabbath as well? Yet, like all God's commandments, the weekly Sabbath rest is for our own good. He told the children of Israel: "Keep the commandments of the Lord, and his statutes, which I command thee this day for thy good" (Deuteronomy 10:13, KJV). And one of those commandments "for thy good" was to rest on the Sabbath day.

God instituted the Sabbath as part of the original Creation week. That is, even before any of the other Ten Commandments existed, the sanctity of the Sabbath rest already did: "Thus the heavens and the earth were finished, and all the host of them. And on the seventh day God ended his work which he had made; and he rested on the seventh day from all his work which he had made. And God blessed the seventh day, and sanctified it: because that in it he had rested from all his work which God created and made" (Genesis 2:1–3, KJV).

The Lord did not originally intend the blessing of the Sabbath just for any one people. He created the day of rest for all humanity, because all people have their origins in the Lord. "God saw that a Sabbath was essential for man, even in Paradise. He needed to lay aside his own interests and pursuits for one day of the seven, that he might more fully contemplate the works of God and meditate upon His power and goodness. He needed a Sabbath to remind him more vividly of God and to awaken gratitude because all that he enjoyed and possessed came from the beneficent hand of the Creator."[3]

Achieving true rest demands much more than merely the physical act of sleeping. Finding rest for our restless minds and bodies requires something beyond putting our heads on our pillows in mindless slumber. It is entering into heaven's Sabbath rest—that is, setting aside the seventh-day Sabbath as the day that God blessed, and then stepping away from all we do, spending time with Him and contemplating what He has done for us. Those who have experienced the peace, the serenity, the joy that comes from anticipating the Sabbath rest and partaking of it week after week, know just how physically, spiritually, and mentally beneficial it can be for work-weary souls.

Choose to Rest

If we aren't careful, the demands on our time can dominate us even to the detriment of our physical, mental, and spiritual health. God has given us two powerful ways to break those vicious cycles of time, two ways to find rest for our restlessness: sleep and the Sabbath. We ourselves can choose to find the rest both of sleep and of the Sabbath. But most of all, heaven longs for us to discover the joy of resting totally, fully, and securely in Jesus, thus experiencing His true rest both now and throughout all eternity.

1. Abraham Joshua Heschel, *The Sabbath* (New York: Farrar, Straus and Giroux, 1979).

2. HealthPeople.gov, "Sleep Health," http://healthypeople.gov/2020/topics-objectives2020/overview.aspx?topicid=38.

3. Ellen G. White, *Patriarchs and Prophets* (Mountain View, Calif.: Pacific Press® Pub. Assn., 1958), 48.

CHAPTER 11

THE HEALING POWER OF FAITH

Faith is a great health restorer: receive it.

For decades researchers have examined the relationship between faith and health. Today we have a mounting body of evidence that faith does make a difference in our total well-being. Faith in a personal God who loves us and only has our best good in mind has a positive impact on both our physical and emotional health. What we believe about God affects every area of our lives. Our spiritual beliefs and practices make a difference in our total well-being. Thus our spiritual lives play a far greater role in determining our overall health than we previously understood.

Although the research is continuing, we clearly realize that faith does matter. Here's a sampling of what researchers have discovered that a dose of spirituality can do for you:

1. Stress: A comprehensive study conducted in Alameda County, California, followed the lifestyle practices of nearly 7,000 Californians. It revealed that West Coast worshippers who participate in church-sponsored activities are markedly less stressed about finances, health, and other daily concerns than nonspiritual individuals.[1]

2. Blood pressure: Senior citizens in a Duke University study who attended religious services, prayed, or read the Bible regularly had lower blood pressure than those who did not follow such practices.[2]

3. Recovery: A Duke University study discovered that devout patients recovering from major surgery spent an average of 11 days in the hospital compared with nonreligious patients, who spent 25 days in the hospital.[3]

4. Immunity: Research on 1,700 adults found that those who attended religious services were less likely to have elevated levels of interleukin-6, an immune substance prevalent in people with chronic diseases.[4]

5. Lifestyle: A review of several studies suggests that spirituality has links with lower suicide rates, less alcohol and drug abuse, less criminal behavior, fewer divorces, and higher marital satisfaction.[5]

6. Depression: Women with "pious" moms are 60 percent less likely to be depressed than those whose mothers aren't so reverent, according to a Columbia University study. Daughters belonging to the same religious denomination as their mothers do are even less likely (71 percent) to suffer the blues while sons are 84 percent less likely.[6]

Wholeness in Brokenness

Faith and spirituality, however, are not all that one needs to have perfect health. Since the arrival of sin, we all suffer to some degree physically, mentally, and spiritually, regardless of how much faith in God we have.

In the Bible, Job, a man of great faith, endured devastating physical ailments. Paul pleaded three times for God to remove his particular thorn in the flesh, but instead of physical healing of his "brokenness," he received a special kind of wholeness: "My grace is sufficient for you," the Lord told him, "for My power is made perfect in weakness" (2 Corinthians 12:9, NIV). No wonder Paul could say, "For when I am weak, then I am strong" (verse 10, NIV).

Such encouragement is particularly meaningful to those who, despite faith, prayer, and medical intervention, still suffer from chronic diseases.

Faith Makes a Difference, but Questions Remain

The research is very convincing: faith does make a difference in our physical as well as our spiritual lives. But significant questions still remain. If we have enough faith, can we live as we please and still be healthy? Does faith give us license to violate the laws of health and still expect to live longer?

Assuming that if you have enough faith your lifestyle choices will make little difference is a misguided presumption that may quickly lead you to end up in the hospital. The idea that faith is some type of magic cure that makes medical professionals unnecessary is a major misunderstanding. Some people believe that if you go to the doctor for a medical problem, you lack faith. They fail to understand that the same God who can heal directly more often guides the skilled medical professionals to accomplish it. *All* healing comes ultimately from God. He is the Great Healer. But *how* He heals and *whom* He uses to accomplish the healing process is up to Him.

Faith Defined and Applied

Let's explore genuine biblical faith, as well as consider its source and results. To understand the meaning of faith, we'll begin with Hebrews 11:1: "Now faith is the substance of things hoped for, the evidence of things not seen" (NKJV).

What is faith, then? It is the substance. The Latin word *substance* comes from two other words: "sub" and "stance." "Sub," of course, means "under." We have words such as *submarine,* a boat that travels under the sea, and *subterranean,* something under the earth. The word *stance* refers to the essence of a thing. The substance is the thing that stands under everything else in your life, supporting, sustaining, and securing it. Faith is the very foundation of our existence.

Standing beneath everything else, it supports all our hopes and sustains us as we grapple with the perplexing questions of life. The essence of a vibrant spiritual life, faith keeps it from crumbling. Abel, Enoch, Noah, Abraham, Jacob, Moses, Joseph, and the other heroes of Hebrews 11 all had one thing in common: faith, a faith that sustained and supported them throughout their lives.

Faith is a relationship with God as a well-known friend, which leads us to do whatever He asks and accept whatever He allows with the absolute assurance that He only wants the best for our lives. It believes that God will strengthen us to triumph over every difficulty and overcome every obstacle until the day we receive our final reward in His eternal kingdom. Thus faith leads you to trust God as someone who loves you, knows what is good for you, and is interested in your happiness.

Energizing our entire being, faith lifts our spirits, encourages our hearts, renews our hope, and changes our vision from what is to what can be. Believing God's promises, it receives His gifts before they even materialize.

Heaven's Hall of Fame

In Hebrews 11, God lists the heroes of faith down through the ages. Their names hang high in heaven's "Hall of Fame." It's surprising that the first example of faith that He gives in Hebrews 11 is of someone who dies without any miraculous deliverance. "By faith Abel offered to God a more excellent sacrifice than Cain, through which he obtained witness that he was righteous, God testifying of his gifts; and through it he being dead still speaks" (Hebrews 11:4, NKJV).

According to the Bible, Abel was a righteous individual. But what was the result of his faith? It got him killed. If he hadn't had faith, he would have lived. Cain did not have faith and lived, while Abel who did have faith, died. That may seem strange to some people who have a mistaken understanding of genuine faith, such as those who believe that if you have enough faith you will always be healed.

Now, let's consider Enoch, the next in Scripture's royal line of faith: "By faith Enoch was translated that he should not see death; and was not found, because God had translated him: for before his translation he had this testimony that he pleased God" (verse 5, KJV).

If Enoch didn't have faith, he would have died. But he did have faith, so he lived. Yet Abel had the same quality of faith and perished. One thing does not puzzle us, however. Each of the worthies of faith in Hebrews 11 teaches us how to trust God. Enoch trusts Him in life, and Abel does so in death.

Now let's look at Noah's example: "By faith Noah being divinely

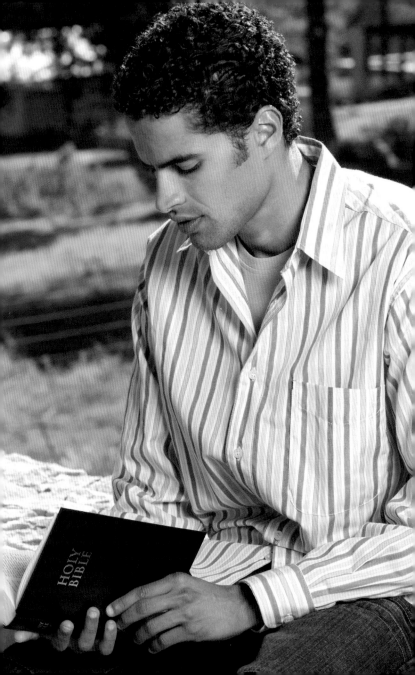

warned of things not yet seen, moved with godly fear, and prepared an ark for the saving of His household" (verse 7, NKJV). His faith led him to do just what God said, even though to the majority of people in his day it must have seemed ridiculous. Obediently Noah followed God's instructions. Trusting Him, he remained where he was for 120 years building an ark despite the fact that there was no rain. Now, that's faith.

Abraham's experience was just the opposite: "By faith Abraham obeyed when he was called to go out to the place which he would afterward receive as an inheritance. And he went out, not knowing where he was going" (verse 8, NKJV). His faith led him to leave the security of his homeland and venture out into the unknown.

What contrasts! Abel died by faith, and Enoch survived by it. Noah stayed by faith, and Abraham ventured out because of it.

Sarah conceived a child by faith when she was 90 years old, and years later Abraham took her son, Isaac, to Mount Moriah at God's command to sacrifice him. There the Lord honored Abraham's faith and delivered the lad. The same God who asked the parents to believe He would give them a child now asked Abraham to believe when He commanded him to sacrifice his son. Of course, God miraculously provided deliverance for Isaac, foreshadowing Jesus' sacrifice and miraculous deliverance of each one of us from the jaws of sin and death.

Here's another contrast found in Hebrews 11. Joseph was faithful to God in spite of the difficult circumstances of his life. As the result of his faithfulness, God honored him. He lived as a witness of the true God amid the wealth and opulence of Egypt. But Moses had the opposite experience. The Lord led him out of Egypt to wander in the wilderness in total dependence on Him. Moses chose to "suffer affliction with the people of God than to enjoy the passing pleasures of sin, esteeming the reproach of Christ greater riches than the treasures in Egypt; for he looked to the reward" (verses 25, 26, NKJV). Joseph had faith and remained in Egypt, while Moses had faith and God told him to leave Egypt. Through faith Joseph became rich, but Moses became poor.

Faith is seeking God's will for my life, whether it's in death as with Abel or in life as with Enoch. Whether it's staying like Noah or going like Abraham, or whether it's living in the luxury of Egypt like Joseph or being a homeless wanderer in the desert like Moses, faith is always an abiding trust in God.

What circumstance do you find yourself in today? Is it facing a life-threatening illness or enjoying good health? Are you perfectly content in your home or anticipating a move and dreading it? Prospering financially or struggling to pay your mortgage? Enjoying a great marriage or finding yourself in a stressful, strained relationship? Do you feel very close to God or distant from Him? Faith, however, is not dependent on our feelings or situations.

Each of the heroes in God's "Hall of Fame" in Hebrews 11 experienced different circumstances in their lives. Faith does not hinge on what's going on around us, but has everything to do with what's going on inside us. Each of the worthies of faith in Hebrews 11 had one common thread running through their lives: they trusted God.

Faith is trusting God for:

- Strength in our weakness
- Hope in our depression
- Guidance in our doubt
- Joy in our sorrow
- Peace in our anxiety
- Wisdom in our ignorance
- Courage in our fear

Not knowing defeat or understanding the word "impossible," faith is filled with courage. Trusting God in all life's circumstances, faith can remain positive whatever happens, because it trusts in the One who knows no defeat. It's that trusting attitude of faith that causes the brain to release positive chemical endorphins, which strengthen the immune system and bring health to our bodies.

Faith's Source

Faith is not some kind of hyped-up positive thinking or self-induced warm feeling. It is not our ability to make ourselves believe something. Hebrews 11:6 describes the source of all faith: "But without faith it is impossible to please Him, for he who comes to God must believe that He is, and that He is a rewarder of those who diligently seek Him" (NKJV).

The source of all faith is an all-powerful, all-knowing, all-loving God. A trusting relationship with the Lord begins with the realization that He loves us and desires only good for us.

Our attitude also plays a significant part in our well-being. It's not just our lifestyle that determines our health. Human emotions also have a significant impact. A study reported by researchers from the University of Kansas found that positive emotions are critical to maintaining good physical health, especially for those deeply impoverished. In other words, if you want to be healthy, you need a positive attitude, particularly if you're enmeshed in difficult circumstances. The study showed that positive emotions such as happiness and contentment are unmistakably linked to better health, even when taking into account a lack of basic needs.

Carol Ryff, psychology professor at the University of Wisconsin–Madison, noted, "There is a science that is emerging that says a positive attitude isn't just a state of mind. It also has linkages to what's going on in the brain and in the body." Ryff has shown that individuals with higher levels of well-being have lower cardiovascular risk, lower levels of stress hormones, and lower levels of inflammation.[7]

God is the source of all positive emotions, and faith taps into those emotions and releases healing power into the body. Faith is trusting God in every circumstance of life, and no other attitude is as life-giving or health-restoring.

Increasing Our Faith

What do you do when your faith is weak? Perhaps you may agree that faith is life-giving, yet feel that you don't have much faith. We have good news for you. You have more faith than you realize. The problem is not that you don't have any faith—it's that you haven't exercised what you have.

In Romans 12:3, Paul says, "As God has dealt to each one a measure of faith" (NKJV). When we make a conscious choice to reach out to our all-loving, all-powerful God and trust Him, He places within our hearts a measure of faith.

Faith is a gift that God gives us. The more we exercise that gift, the more it will grow. As we learn to trust Him amid the trials and challenges we face in life, our faith increases. Sometimes our moments of greatest desperation are those of our greatest growth in faith.

We can also expand our faith as we meditate upon God's Word. As the truths of the Bible fill our minds, our faith increases rapidly. The Scriptures affirm this divine reality in Paul's letter to the Romans: "So then faith comes by hearing, and hearing by the word of God" (Romans 10:17, NKJV).

The more we saturate our minds with Scripture, the greater our faith will be. His Word dispels our doubts. Would you like to open your heart to God and by faith receive His power today? If you desire to enter into a new relationship of trust and confidence in God, you can ask Him to give you a trusting heart so that you can experience the health benefits of a living faith.

---

1. David N. Elkins, "Spirituality," *Psychology Today*, September 1, 1999, http://psychologytoday.com/articles/199909/spirituality.

2. Ibid.

3. Ibid.

4. Ibid.

5. Ibid.

6. Ibid.

7. Quoted in Sharon Jayson, "Power of a Super Attitude," *USA Today*, October 12, 2004, http://usatoday30.usatoday.com/news/health/2004-10-12-mind-body_x.htm.

Contributors and Consultants

Albert Reece
Physician

Allan Handysides
Physician

Benjamin Carson
Neurosurgeon

Clifford Goldstein
Writer

Delbert W. Baker
Theologian

Duane McBride
Sociologist

Fred Hardinge
Registered Dietitian

Katia Reinert
Nurse Practitioner

Mark A. Finley
Pastor

Gary Fraser
Researcher

Gary Hopkins
Researcher

Peter N. Landless
Physician

Neil Nedley
Physician

Heather Quintana
Vibrant Life Editor

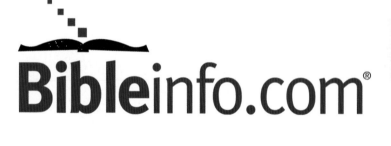

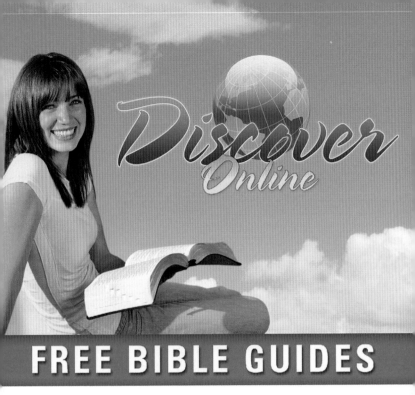

FREE BIBLE GUIDES

It's easy to learn more about the Bible!

Request: www.biblestudies.com/request

Write: Discover
P.O. Box 999
Loveland, CO 80539

Call: 1-888-456-7933

Study Online: www.bibleschools.com

Offering **God's good news** for a better life
today and for eternity

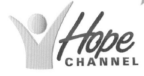

hopetv.org

Christian television programing about faith, health, relationships, and community